A DECENT PROPOSAL

For Ann, James, David and Kathryn – DME

For Janet, Jeremy and Harry – HME

A DECENT PROPOSAL
Ethical Review of Clinical Research

Donald Evans and Martyn Evans

Centre for Philosophy and Health Care
University of Wales Swansea, UK

JOHN WILEY & SONS
Chichester · New York · Brisbane · Toronto · Singapore

Copyright © 1996 by John Wiley & Sons Ltd,
Baffins Lane, Chichester,
West Sussex PO19 1UD, England

National   01243 779777
International (+44) 1243 779777

Other Wiley Editorial Offices

John Wiley & Sons, Inc., 605 Third Avenue,
New York, NY 10158-0012, USA

Jacaranda Wiley Ltd, 33 Park Road, Milton,
Queensland 4064, Australia

John Wiley & Sons (Canada) Ltd, 22 Worcester Road,
Rexdale, Ontario M9W 1L1, Canada

John Wiley & Sons (Asia) Pte Ltd, 2 Clementi Loop #02-01,
Jin Xing Distripark, Singapore 0512

Library of Congress Cataloging-in-Publication Data

Evans, Donald, *1939–*
    A decent proposal : ethical review of clinical research / Donald
Evans and Martyn Evans.
        p. cm.
    Includes bibliographical references and index.
    ISBN 0-471-96334-8 (cased)
        1. Human experimentation in medicine—Moral and ethical aspects.
    2. Peer review of research grant proposals.   3. Research ethics.
    4. Ethics committees.   I. Evans, Martyn, *1956–* .   II. Title.
    R853.H8E87   1996
    174′.28—dc20   95–46949
                                                                CIP

British Library Cataloguing in Publication Data

A catalogue record for this book is available from the British Library

ISBN 0-471-96334-8

Produced from camera-ready copy supplied by the authors
Printed and bound in Great Britain by Biddles Ltd, Guildford and King's Lynn

This book is printed on acid-free paper responsibly manufactured from sustainable forestation, for which
at least two trees are planted for each one used for paper production.

Contents

Preface

This book is an attempt to describe in plain language the concerns, responsibilities, general issues and particular pitfalls facing members of research ethics committees. We have written it in the hope that it will help many such committee members to feel better prepared for the job that they have been asked to do in carrying out ethical review of clinical research – and, just as importantly, that it will help many clinical researchers to have a clearer appreciation for themselves of how ethically-appropriate research protects their research subjects. The more that clinical researchers and the ethics committees that review their proposals appreciate each other's concerns, the more likely it is that research subjects can be protected by the positive means of sound research design, rather than by the negative means of rejection of unacceptable proposals.

As academic philosophers by profession, we occasionally come across the view that philosophy is a remote, obscure, impenetrable discipline with few if any practical uses. Perhaps sometimes academic philosophy really is like that; but we think that in terms of the contribution which university teaching can make to the life of the community, practical reasoning in plain language holds as honourable a place as scholarly theorising. Ten years spent teaching philosophy to health care professionals have convinced us of the value of bringing practical moral problems and philosophical reflection together. Almost as much time spent serving on research ethics committees has convinced us of how frequently medical professionals and laypeople alike feel under-prepared for the job they are asked to do. So in this book we shall try to bring our practical understanding of philosophical reflection to bear on some of the real and important moral challenges to which modern, scientific health care continually gives rise.

Whilst relatively few people actually conduct clinical research, any of us might at any time become ill or injured and find ourselves in the rôle of patient; and almost any patient might be an appropriate subject for some clinical research or other. Knowing this gives a keener edge to the otherwise perhaps rather abstract responsibilities facing members of research ethics committees. It has certainly influenced our approach to our own service on research ethics committees, whether as committee chairman, vice-chairman or ordinary member. We have learned how important it is to try to combine the perspective of the ordinary patient with the different kinds of specialist expertise which research ethics committees need. As medical laymen ourselves we have appreciated and respected those who provide the scientific knowledge that we lack; but at the same time we have remained aware that in moral judgement there are no experts as such, and that medical or scientific knowledge is not in itself a source of moral reflection. Being a moral philosopher does not make anyone an expert in moral judgement either; if there are any 'courses' in becoming morally better or morally wiser people, those courses will not be found in universities. But philosophy does consist in sustained, critical reasoning about the ideas and claims with which we are all bombarded in daily life – and making a habit of this can in its turn make us more careful, consistent and critical in both drawing up and scrutinising research proposals, something from which the ethical review of clinical research can only benefit.

We have tried to bring such a habit to bear upon our own review of the many clinical research proposals which we have studied over the years, and upon the part we have played in Committee discussions and decisions. Most of all, then, this book draws on the experience of reviewing and discussing such research proposals, and on the experience of sharing with lay and medical colleagues alike the challenges of adjudicating on them. We hope to be able to convey that experience in a way that will be readily accessible to committee members and to clinical researchers alike, and that in the following pages they will recognise not merely the concerns which trouble them but also the kind of reflection that can make those concerns more manageable.

Swansea, December 1995

Acknowledgements

This book initially began in work towards a research project undertaken in 1992 for, and with the generous support of, the UK government's Department of Health. We are indebted to the Department of Health for that opportunity. We owe a great debt also the members and chairpersons of West Glamorgan Research Ethics Committee, Mid Glamorgan District Ethics Committee, and Simbec Research's Independent Ethics Committee for the opportunity for us to gain the experiences which have stimulated and informed this book. We have greatly benefitted from working with colleagues in the Centre for Philosophy and Health Care, University of Wales Swansea and in the Association of Independent Clinical Research Contractors in the development and presentation of an annual programme of national training conferences on good practice for members of research ethics committees. Much of the preparation of this book was made possible by the generosity of the University of Wales Swansea in granting to Martyn Evans a period of research leave in the Spring of 1994, and by the corresponding generosity of the Ersta Institute of Health Care Ethics, Stockholm, Sweden, who provided academic facilities and support through a Visiting Scholarship for that period.

Helpful advice was provided at an early stage by the comments of an anonymous referee for John Wiley & Sons, and throughout by our Editor Verity Waite and Senior Production Editor Lewis Derrick. Among the many other individuals whose comments and advice have helped us we must particularly mention Dr. John Dewhurst, Dr. Peter Dewland, Mr. Simon Emery, Dr. David Greaves, Dr. Søren Holm, Dr. Richard Nicholson, Dr. David Powell, Mr. Tom Russell, Ms. Kate Walker and Mr. Alan Willson.

We have made extensive use of lighthearted quotations in the text, and in tracking down their original appearances we were invaluably helped by Mr. Rupert Jarvis. We are indebted to Tessa LeBars Management for the extract from *Hancock* ('The Blood Donor') written by Ray Galton and Alan Simpson (used on p.46 in this volume); to Peters, Fraser and Dunlop and to Macintyre Management for the extract from *Blackadder II*, written by Richard Curtis and Ben Elton (p.91); to David Wilkinson Associates for the extract from *Fawlty Towers*, written by John

Cleese and Connie Booth (p.168); and to Kay-Gee-Bee Music Ltd. for the extract from 'The Philosopher's Song' from *Monty Python's Flying Circus* (p.78). The quotation from the *Observer* newspaper (p.37 in this volume) was taken from L.Susan Stebbings, *Thinking to Some Purpose*, published by Penguin Books in 1939. A number of other quotations were culled from Ned Sherrin's *Oxford Dictionary of Humorous Quotations*, published by Oxford University Press in 1995. We are grateful to Oxford University Press for their assistance and cooperation. The original appearances of the extracts in question were as follows: the quotation from Oliver Edwards (p.41 in this volume) appeared in George Birkbeck Hill's edition of Boswell's *Life of Samuel Johnson*, Clarendon Press, 1934; from Alan Bennett (p.51) in his *Getting on* in *Forty Years On and Other Plays*, Faber, 1991; from F.M. Cornford (p.53) in his *Microcosmographia Academica*, 10th. edn., Mainsail Press, 1993; from Ed Gardner (p.65) in *Duffy's Tavern*, a 1940s U.S. radio programme; from Oliver Herford (p.72) in his *The Entirely New Cynic's Calendar*, Paul Elder, 1905; from Judith Martin (p.90) in her *Miss Manners' Guide to Rearing Perfect Children*, Hamilton, 1985; from H.H.Munro (p.98) in his *Reginald in Russia: The Baker's Dozen* in *Penguin Complete Saki*, Penguin, 1982; from Alan Clarke M.P. (p.112) in his *Diaries*, Weidenfield and Nicolson, 1993; from Christopher Fry (p.124) in his *The Lady's not for Burning: a Comedy*, Oxford University Press, 1950; from Gwyn Thomas (p.163) in *Punch*, 18th. June 1950; from the Chancellor, the Rt. Hon. Kenneth Clarke M.P. (p.178) in an after dinner speech given on 9th March 1989, when Secretary of State for Health, to the Royal College of General Practitioners; from Neil Simon (p.207) in his *The Gingerbread Lady* in *Collected Plays of Neil Simon*, Volume II, Random House, 1979; and again from Alan Bennett (p.210) in his *Habeus Corpus* in *Forty Years On and Other Plays*, Faber, 1991.

Finally of course our biggest debts are to our families whose support and understanding has made it possible for us to attempt this work at all. To them we are enduringly grateful.

Chapter One

Why ethical review? The moral context of clinical research

1.1   The development of ethical review

Never be a pioneer. It's the early Christian that gets the fattest lion.
(Saki)

1.1.1   The origins of formalised ethical review

Formalised ethical review of medical research has developed only since the
Second World War.   Indeed it did not really begin to mushroom into
today's complex and varied activity until the 1970s. This development has
coincided with an explosion in clinical research activity. This is most
obvious in the area of the development of new medicines where hundreds
of thousands of research subjects are now used each year in the clinical
development stage of pharmaceutical products.   It was in response to
specific cases of the mistreatment of human subjects of medical research
that ethical review was formalised.   The quickest progress in the
development of ethical review happened in the United States where the
system quickly acquired the backing of statutory authority.   Elsewhere,
until relatively recently, ethical review has generally been conducted on the
basis of guidelines and advice from various professional and governmental
authorities without the force of the law.   The United Kingdom is the
clearest example of a major player in medical research which has adopted
this approach. In section 13.1 of this book we will discuss whether legal
backing is desirable for ethical review of research on human subjects. But

first it is worth briefly mapping out how ethical review developed in these two countries in order to appreciate the value of the activity and the rôle it has played and will continue to play in the widening world of human subject research.

Of course ethical review has developed to varying degrees in many other countries and is currently the subject of considerable concern in the European Union, which is pursuing a harmonisation of standards in clinical research[1]. Some countries have known a mix of statutory and non-statutory review. For example, in Denmark a previously non-statutory system was given the full backing of the law in 1992, making it a criminal offence to carry out research on human subjects without the approval of a properly constituted ethical review committee[2]. Many Central European countries are also busy developing ethical review mechanisms following the recent political changes.

It would be a mistake to think that before formal ethical review procedures were introduced no attention had been paid to the safety and interests of medical research subjects. Perhaps the most notable example of an individual researcher showing such concern was Walter Reed in his production of a consent form for subjects in yellow fever experiments in 1900. This form acknowledged the risks the subjects faced in agreeing to take part in the research and it recorded their willingness to face them. By contrast it was the **lack** of consent, combined with the inhumane procedures involved, that condemned much of the supposedly medical research carried out by Nazi doctors as being instead crimes against humanity. For example, many subjects in this 'research' were forced to act as cultures for typhus and malaria to test vaccines. Twenty-three doctors were convicted at the Nuremberg trials and the exposure of their deeds led to adoption of the first internationally recognised code of medical ethics – the Nuremberg Code – which highlighted the need for proper consent, the avoidance of unnecessary physical and mental suffering and the prohibition of unnecessary and aimless research. The rights of research subjects were also highlighted in the Code, most notable amongst them being the right of any research subject to withdraw from a trial or study at any time.

1.1.2   A statutory system[3]

It took some time for this Code to be implemented in terms of formal surveillance of research on human subjects. In 1953 a non-medical behavioural research project into jury practice in the United States of

America involved secret surveillance of jurors in their deliberations. In 1955 this was exposed in a U.S. Senate Committee and led to demands for respect for the rights of all subjects in behavioural research. The establishment of the National Institutes of Health research hospital saw a call for all human subject research to be reviewed by committees of medical experts. However, it took the serious adverse events in the experimental use of thalidomide in the United States to bring about statutory control of ethical review of medical research. The Federal Food, Drug and Cosmetic Act of 1938 allowed doctors to test such drugs without ethical review. In 1962 this Act was amended in the light of the damage caused to foetuses by thalidomide and for the first time anywhere in the world the informed consent of research subjects was officially demanded in Congressional legislation affecting all subjects of research involving experimental drugs. Even so, experimentation without informed consent continued, and the injection of live cancer cells into feeble and seriously ill patients in research on the immune system in 1963 led to a lawsuit and to severe criticism of medical research activity. The Director of the National Institutes of Health, set up a committee to examine the system of ethical review; in 1966 this led the Surgeon General to insist that all publicly funded research be reviewed by independent ethical committees.

But further shocks were to come when in 1972 the Alabama study of syphilis was uncovered. This study of three hundred black syphilis sufferers had been running since 1932. It was designed to study the natural history of the disease and denied information and treatment to the sufferers, even after the advent of penicillin. Reaction to this study, which became known as the 'Tuskegee Study', resulted in the National Research Act Public Law 93-348, July 12, 1974. Section 474 demanded the setting up of Institutional Review Boards to review all publicly funded biomedical and behavioural research involving human subjects. This was demanded 'in order to protect the rights of human subjects of such research'. Since that time a National Commission for the Protection of Human Subjects of Biomedical and Behavioral Research has been set up, with responsibility for guidance and advice on ethical review of research; additionally, various federal regulations governing ethical review of research have been produced.

1.1.3   A non-statutory system

In the United Kingdom the thalidomide tragedy also played an important rôle. It led the Medical Research Council to make a statement in its annual report (1962-3) about 'Responsibility in investigations on human subjects'[4]. The Declaration of Helsinki in 1964 added weight to the discussion of ethical review of clinical research[5]. Thereafter for some years the Royal College of Physicians took the lead in promoting ethical review of clinical research in the United Kingdom. It issued reports in 1967 and 1973 making various recommendations for the setting up of ethical review committees in all clinical research institutions, and it made various suggestions about the structure of such committees. The U.K. government Department of Health and Social Security produced its own guidance in accordance with these suggestions in 1975[6]. However the resulting system of review was extremely varied in quality and its extent was not known even to the Department itself, which did not hold complete records of the identity or whereabouts of the active review committees. It was known that in some areas such committees had not been set up and there was need for further reform of the system[7].

In 1991 a revised set of guidelines was issued by the Department of Health[8] at which time all Research Ethics Committees (RECs) were to be reconstituted and conform to the Department's pattern. These guidelines instructed Health Authorities to set up such committees, but the instructions had no statutory backing. (Hereafter for convenience we will refer to this Document simply as the *Guidelines*.) Since 1991 there has been a good deal of discussion about the efficiency and effectiveness of this system, especially with respect to the review of multi-centre protocols. We ourselves hope to contribute to this discussion in Chapter Twelve. Further reviews of the system are believed to be imminent.

We'll see in later chapters that there is a small element of statutory ethical review in the United Kingdom system, in the form of regulatory control. Even so, there is no criminalisation of improper research on human subjects beyond the provisions of the common law. There have been calls to provide statutory backing to the ethical review procedure in the United Kingdom[9] but there is little prospect of such control being introduced in the foreseeable future.

1.2   The utilitarian tradition

> *Hain't we got all the fools in town on our side? And*
> *ain't that a big enough majority in any town?*
> (Mark Twain)

Most of this book is concerned with the moral restraints to be put upon clinical research;   we will see that the first task of RECs is to make sure that these restraints are understood and observed. But we should not let this primary concern obscure the fact that there is a general moral case in favour of conducting clinical research, and that one reason why the restraints are important is because clinical research is itself morally important. The importance of clinical research stems from its beneficial consequences, and the moral tradition which most clearly emphasises the importance of beneficial consequences is Utilitarianism. Because it seems to offer a ready-made moral framework for the pursuit of medical progress, we shall in this section consider the claims of Utilitarianism – and look at some of its limitations. In the following section we will appreciate how those limitations largely define both the purpose of ethical review and the proper moral concerns of RECs. For the attempt to make medically advantageous use of the human body in research forces us to reconcile two competing considerations: on the one hand the need to obtain the maximum practical benefits in terms of therapeutic advance, and on the other hand the need to preserve due respect for people's individual safety, dignity and freedom of choice.

There is no doubt that we make use of other people – and other people's bodies – in many ways. The precedents for doing this are well established: think of manual labour, for instance. Medical research is in this sense just another way in which people may make use of each other; the moral challenges of finding an appropriate regulatory framework for medical research could be compared to the job of finding other such frameworks in areas of public interest, such as employment law and housing law. At a very general level, law and policy on these matters aim at maximising the public benefits to be obtained from any chosen course; historically, the drive to maximise benefits has been given expression in the moral theory known as Utilitarianism. Of all moral theories, and indeed of all theoretical philosophical positions, Utilitarianism is the most widely known. There are very good reasons for this: first, there is something intuitively appealing about the idea that morality consists in 'doing as much good as possible', particularly so long as the meaning of 'good' is left conveniently vague and unspecified. Second, utilitarian arguments are to a large extent **public interest** arguments. They hinge on showing that the public benefits of a particular course of action are both significant (they are worth our while pursuing) and real (they are very likely to be produced). And on the face of it, everyone has an interest in the production of real and significant public benefits. Third, Utilitarianism evolved as a theoretical justification for liberal public welfare reforms that have produced many of the social protections now taken for granted in modern states[10]. Political arguments about the shape of public policy are characteristically couched in terms of what will produce the greatest public benefits overall: the popular language of Utilitarianism is a natural vehicle for debate over public policy. It seems equally natural to begin a justification for the practice of conducting medical research on human subjects by appealing to the characteristically Utilitarian considerations of ultimate greatest benefit.   For instance, consider this passage from the the British Paediatric Association's *Guidelines for the Ethical Conduct of Medical Research Involving Children*, revised and reissued in 1992:

> Medical research involving children is an important means of promoting child health and wellbeing.... Research with children is worthwhile, if each project:
>
> - has an identifiable prospect of benefit to children;
> - is well designed and well conducted;
> - does not simply duplicate earlier work;
> - is not undertaken primarily for financial or professional advantage;
> - involves a statistically appropriate number of subjects;
> - and eventually is to be properly reported.[11]

It is striking that such a morally sensitive subject as the use of children in medical research is approached, first of all, by a robust emphasis on the good that can be done.   The passage quoted takes it for granted that the bedrock of morally acceptable research is that the research be worthwhile;   and in pretty well any context, the obvious interpretation of 'worthwhile' refers to the production of end results.   The clear point of each of the listed characteristics of worthwhile research is that they contribute to the effective production of results (this is true even of the warning about conducting research for financial or professional advantage).   In effect, the claim runs, what makes research on children a good thing is just the good things that we hope will be produced by it;   and these good things consist in the promotion of children's health and well-being.   And after all, who could deny that there is a compelling public interest in the health and well-being of our children?

This is a highly plausible claim;   the only problem with it is that as a specification of morally acceptable research it seems incomplete.   Almost everyone would want to make some important additions to the list of qualifications given above, if they were to turn it from a specification of a worthwhile **project** into an account of an acceptable **practice** – that is to say, almost everyone would want to insist on proper protections for the children on whom the research was to be conducted.   Indeed, the British Paediatric Association go on to add precisely these kinds of qualifications – making their absence from the definition of 'worthwhile' research more apparent[12].   Now this addition is crucial, as is the distinction between a project (which we generally picture in terms of the goals we want to achieve at its end) and a practice (which we generally picture in terms of the sorts of things that are done in it).   An example might make this clearer: we could easily approve the project of searching for a well tolerated all-purpose cytotoxic drug, yet virtually everyone would condemn the practice of conducting that search by testing the tolerability of promising drugs on healthy volunteers.

The distinction between 'project' and 'practice' – in the way we have defined them here – goes to the heart of a further distinction concerning what the term 'utilitarian' can mean; there are two senses of the term which, while superficially similar, are ultimately so different as to reflect irreconcilable views about morality in general, and about the morality of practices such as medical research in particular. This might have been nothing more than an academic philosophical distinction if it weren't for the fact that the term 'utilitarian' is in reasonably common use, or for the fact that it appears to be the name of an intuitively reasonable way of thinking about public policy. Because of this, we ought to be as clear about the distinction as we can.

Briefly, it is this: one of the two senses of 'utilitarian' is a loose, colloquial and relaxed one, in which there is room to consider both ends and means (and therefore both projects and practices); the other is a strict, technical and rigidly demanding one, in which there is room to consider only ultimate ends (and therefore only projects). The colloquial conception of a utilitarian view means little more than having a special concern for the consequences of actions or policies, arranging them, as far as possible, to produce the most benefit for the most people in the long run. To the extent that public policies are conceived basically with the aim of producing the most widespread, long-run benefits, they are inevitably utilitarian in this loose sense; and to the extent that we appreciate them for their benefits (or condemn them for their failure) then we judge as utilitarians – again, in this loose sense. But whilst this concern is certainly also true of the strict sense of a utilitarian view, it stops short of the key features of the formal theory of Utilitarianism. These key features are threefold, as follows.

First, Utilitarianism assumes that absolutely any and all consequences can in principle be measured, compared and aggregated together in the common coinage of how much good they achieve or how much harm they avoid. So for example, the industrial benefits of finding a cure for the common cold are assumed to be measurable by the same yardstick as, for example, the individual benefits of genetic manipulations to correct Huntingdon's Disease. Second, Utilitarianism assumes that we can – indeed must – work out which courses of action will lead to the best positive balance of benefit over harm, taking into account all the consequences of all the available alternative courses of action open to us. So if the cure for the common cold led to greater structural unemployment through higher industrial productivity, then that consequence would be an obligatory part of the ultimate total, possibly tipping the balance against releasing and distributing the new therapy. Finally, Utilitarianism ultimately disregards the way in which harms and benefits are distributed: all that counts is the achievement of the best possible total, even if *en route* to a general improvement for the many, a few people are grievously disadvantaged. If, therefore, the research programme for a well tolerated all-purpose cytotoxic drug temporarily ran out of patient-subjects and could proceed only by using healthy subjects, then Utilitarianism would sanction, indeed require, us to use them so long as the morbidity and mortality involved did not outweigh the benefits of the programme's successful conclusion.

These two senses of 'utilitarian' are therefore crucially distinct. We can see that the more casual concern with the general idea of maximising benefits fits very well with ordinary, commonsense, practical morality. At the same time a little reflection shows us that a strict insistence on the 'countability' and 'gradeability' of widely differing kinds of benefits and harms fits very badly with our experience of life's variety and unpredictability – and, what's more, very badly with our moral intuitions about the protection of individuals.

To take the problem of 'countability' first, no doubt we do indeed try to make life as orderly and predictable as we can; but equally there is no doubt that this is an uphill struggle against the limitations of our knowledge and the volatility of our own and others' desires and motives. We can look ahead a little way, but we cannot see very far, and any theory requiring us to have long-range vision of the consequences of our actions is going to be implausible and unconvincing. This is a **practical** difficulty for Utilitarianism, since no humanly realistic moral judgement is going to have the long-range, comprehensive scope that the theory requires. The style of the colloquial utilitarian perspective is well suited to the morality of large-scale actions and policies which will affect the public good: innovations and changes in state provision and regulation, welfare, criminal and civil law, and so on. But as an account of individual moral judgements within relatively closed areas of responsibility, the obligation to count up remote or long-range consequences seems unrecognisable. No overworked physician, for instance, either could or should try to decide to distribute her time between demanding patients, on the basis of working out which patient's early recovery would be accompanied by the maximum additional benefits to his worried family, hard-pressed colleagues, or impatient employer.

Worse is to come, however, since this practical difficulty is firmly eclipsed by a **theoretical** difficulty concerning the 'gradeability' of different benefits and harms. As we shall see further in section 5.5, there is something essentially confused about the attempt to measure different kinds of consequences by the same yardstick. We think the attempt is confused because it relies on reducing different kinds of consequences to a single kind: and this means converting the entire range of human values – from courage, dignity, generosity, freedom, equality, fraternity and tolerance to beauty, delicacy, tenderness, reverence, awe and humility, not to mention sweetness, savouriness, astringency or the 'reaching of parts that other beers cannot reach' – to a single value, utility. In plain terms, it seems obvious that we can weigh or measure together only those things which are comparable, that is, which really are (or really can be reduced to) the same sort of thing. Were the Utilitarian publicly to try and weigh in the same scales such wildly contrasting outcomes as the number of new houses built, your success in an examination, reductions in the birth rate, my sadness at the loss of a relative, improvements in peri-operative pain control, an extra penny on the standard rate of income tax, the genetic manipulation of a raspberry with a fuller flavour or the appearance of the fifth edition of this book, then he would face derision. The trouble is that precisely this absurdity lies at the heart of any theory which rests on the reduction of all values to a single one.

Modern utilitarians recognise the problem, and some have tried to limit it by confining the scope of their theory to the most narrow range of consequences, usually in a specific area of application, for instance the idea of 'welfare' – which is already varied enough, covering as it does such areas as housing, education, health, or social security[13]. Further ingenious refinements, mostly concerned with tying the idea of benefit or utility to people's expressions of **preferences**, have been put forward[14]. Whilst they have the unfortunate effect of making Utilitarianism much less like Utilitarianism, as it were, they do improve its plausibility when it is brought to bear upon fairly close alternative policies on a specific matter. Different outcomes can sometimes be compared for their impact on large, undifferentiated numbers of people, as when for instance one particular route for a new motorway is compared to an alternative route a few miles to the south. The kinds of effects involved will be similar in both cases – noise, disruption and so forth. If significantly different numbers of people are affected in the two options, and no other important distinguishing factors can be identified, then the choice of the route affecting fewer people can plausibly be expressed in Utilitarian terms. But it is much more difficult for the Utilitarian to describe the decision to invest in motorways rather than in railways, or to describe the case for spending money on roadbuilding rather than on a programme of energy research, or urban renewal schemes, or increased overseas aid.

This is another reason why, ultimately, Utilitarianism cannot **on its own terms** give a respectable justification for conducting medical research on human subjects, because to specify the alternative uses of the resources involved – resources which must include the time, inconvenience and perhaps distress of the subjects themselves – would be an endless task. What's more, even if it could be achieved there is no earthly reason to suppose that the alternatives would be anything like so closely comparable as alternative motorway routes.

Since the problems of comparison largely stem from the fact that our different kinds of values just are so irreducibly different, we might now wonder why it is that anyone would try to condense all our values into a single one in this way. The answer seems to be that Utilitarianism tries to provide a theory of right action, a theory which will both show us what we ought to do and account for why we ought to do it. We ought to do whatever produces the greatest net balance of benefit over harm, and the reason that we ought to do this is simply that this **is** what morally right action is to consist in. In other words, Utilitarianism claims to give us a definition of 'the good' in terms of the maximal production of benefits. Since all our various values, moral, social, aesthetic and so forth, consist in different forms of 'the good', Utilitarianism must attempt to explain them all. Obviously, then, it must try to do so in terms of the production of benefits. But if the explanations are to be the same in all cases, then the benefits must be strictly comparable, indeed, interchangeable. And what this comes to is a reduction of all forms of positively valued consequences to a single kind, that is, consequences which exhibit a single kind of positive value which is benefit, or utility.

The superficial appeal of this reasoning is easy to see, and has probably been felt at some time by most students of moral thought. From a Utilitarian perspective, the ends really do justify the means, because there simply are no other kinds of justification. It follows that any moral objections to a course of action approved by a Utilitarian calculation must be an objection to Utilitarianism itself, since Utilitarianism claims to account for all moral judgements. The trouble is that the weakness of the claim is just as obvious: for we want to know how it is that certain kinds of outcomes can be picked out as beneficial and others as harmful, without appealing to some independent scale of values. Simply to assert that some consequences produce benefit and others produce harm won't do: for one thing, people disagree over whether particular outcomes really are beneficial, and for another, people disagree over whether it is justifiable to produce an advantage for the many at the expense of the few. Utilitarianism is ultimately unable to explain these disagreements. For instance, it can't explain the moral wrongness – which virtually everyone would nevertheless recognise – of establishing the maximum tolerance levels of a successful cytotoxic drug on healthy subjects. And if we can't agree on what marks out the good from the bad outcomes, we can't even begin to measure and compare different outcomes in the way that Utilitarianism requires.

If Utilitarianism can't explain the relative moral value of different consequences, then neither can it account for the variety of different kinds of – and often competing – values. The moral wrongness of sacrificing healthy subjects to the pursuit of important clinical breakthroughs lies partly in the importance of respecting the rights and dignity of individuals, and partly in the importance of justice: here it is obvious that other senses of 'the good', not credibly explained by Utilitarianism, are at work.

Despite these criticisms, it is worth our spending time considering Utilitarianism because of: (i) its historical influence in matters of public policy; (ii) its echoes in popular moral thought; (iii) its superficial conformity with commonsense practical moral reasoning; (iv) its apparent suitability for describing the imperative to pursue research; and (v) its providing the background or contrast to all the considerations which make us pause and review clinical research – all the considerations, in short, which should occupy the REC, and which we shall be exploring in the coming chapters. First let's conclude our opening chapter with a concrete illustration of how modern liberal society – the natural home of the REC – finally rejects Utilitarian thought in favour of individual freedom and protection.

1.3   Individual and social responsibilities

Cannot come [stop] Lie follows [stop]
(telegram recalled by Marcel Proust)

It is pretty evident that when we need medical treatment we want it to be the best available, and that we hope to benefit from the cumulative processes of medical research. In this we stand on the shoulders of previous patients who were the subjects of research in the past: without them, it is more than likely that we could not now receive the treatments we need, or at least that we could not do so with any confidence as to the safety and desirability of those treatments. So it seems right to ask whether, as patients (or even as ordinary citizens who are merely potential patients), we have any obligations towards future patients, in terms of enabling the cumulative process of research to continue in order that existing treatments be improved and new ones developed.

Again, most of us expect to receive these treatments more or less as of right, perhaps (though not necessarily) in virtue of the tax and national insurance contributions paid by us or our close relatives. However, we should distinguish between on the one hand a 'right' (if indeed it be a right) to receive the best treatment which is as a matter of fact available, and on the other hand a 'right' to expect that best treatment to be continously developed and improved, where this requires more research to be done on patients. It is hard to think that we could as individuals oblige other people to take part in medical research on our behalf. Certainly any such expectations that we might have should be mirrored by their expectations of us. Perhaps, then, there are mutual expectations of this kind - or, to put the point in more familiar terms, might we have obligations to society to be willing to take part in medical research?

Rights and responsibilities go together: logically speaking, any rights that we hold will obviously require other people to behave in certain ways towards us. But morally speaking, we may feel that we have to 'earn' at least some of our rights, by behaving responsibly and by contributing to the social pool of benefits, experience and expertise from which the various entitlements are drawn by ourselves and others. The utilitarian tradition, which we discussed in the last section, although using different language is essentially concerned with the same problems. Society can provide benefits for its members, including the benefits of health care, only to the extent that its members contribute to the social pool. The question then arises as to what kinds of responsibilities we have: should our social contributions be obligatory or merely voluntary?

There is no doubt that some of them are obligatory: if our earnings are sufficient then we cannot legally avoid paying tax and national insurance contributions. Wage-earners simply have to pay for the social provision of health care. This remains true regardless of whether they themselves or their families will ever call on that provision as patients. But there is equally no doubt that taking part in medical research is meant to be voluntary, and we may wonder why this is so. A case could be made, in other words, for regarding it as a part of our mandatory social responsibilities that we take part in (suitably designed and properly safeguarded) medical research, should the need arise, possibly in the ordinary course of receiving medical attention, treatment and aftercare. The case would consist very largely in noticing, as we did above, that we already benefit from existing research, and that we wish and expect to benefit both now and in the future from the continuous development of medical knowledge. The case might be bolstered by reactions against the prevailing ideology of the 1980s, in which social considerations and a sense of social responsibility were generally subordinated to the desires and expectations of the individual, very often in frankly consumerist terms. In health care ethics, the fashion for making individual autonomy the dominant moral consideration has begun to subside, and indeed to attract hostile criticism[15]. The case for obliging us to participate in medical research would emphasise the perils of sacrificing our sense of community on the altar of individual freedom of choice.

Objections to the case for obligatory participation in research need not be made in terms of individualism, however. There is a tradition in morals of distinguishing between those responsibilities which we can be required to meet, and those which we cannot. We require people to be truthful, but we admire those who are brave and self-sacrificing; we condemn those who are dishonest, but we sympathise with those who are just unable to be heroes. Thus, a society can work if enough people are honest, but it can excel if some people are virtuous beyond this. Following this, it is presumably a better thing for society if at least some of our social responsibilities are met voluntarily, out of a sense of solidarity and altruism. Indeed, this is the dominant view in blood and tissue donation, and these procedures are almost always praised in terms of the generosity and social solidarity on which they rely, and, we might suppose, which they inspire. The assumption would then be that undergoing medical research is more like these activities than it is like paying income tax. (If this is so, it will also be something to do with the fact that medical research procedures are likely to interfere with our bodily integrity – something which is respected and protected by law in ordinary clinical care, where it is we and not future patients who stand to benefit from what is done.)

Although a case for obligatory participation in medical research could be made, then, it has certainly not been generally found to be convincing; as things stand, the choice of whether or not to take part in medical research is, in liberal countries, intended to remain firmly the prerogative of the individual patient. Indeed, as we shall see, the voluntariness of participation in research is held to be so important as to constitute one of the two central concerns of RECs, and one of the two key respects in which the research subject's interests must be protected.

We have seen in this chapter that the quest for medical progress has on occasion involved risky and sometimes reckless use of both patients and healthy subjects, in experiments that have not always been of scientific value. Leaving aside bad science, we have recognised that it is in the nature of valuable medical research that there is likely to be some risk to the subjects on whom it is conducted, if for no other reason than that the outcomes of any genuine research are to some extent unknown at the time when the research is begun. Even where well conceived research has led to undoubted advances in medical knowledge, we have seen that the utilitarian view, that such advances will in the long run justify severe or unauthorised harms to research subjects now, cannot be reconciled with the respect which we feel we owe morally to each other as individual members of society. And even the more modest view, that participating in properly safeguarded research should be a mandatory part of our normal social obligations such as paying income tax, does not hold sway at the present time.

Taken together, these considerations reveal the research subject who is centre-stage in medical research as being a vulnerable volunteer. If that description is correct, then we need no further reasons for thinking him to need and deserve appropriate respect and protection. This is the central task of ethical review, and of the REC in particular, and we shall turn now to examining this task in more detail.

Notes

1   This is evidenced by the publication of *Guidelines and Recommendations for European Ethics Committees*, Brussels: European Forum for Good Clinical Practice (June 1995).

2   See Holm, S., 'How many members can you have in your IRB? - An overview of the Danish System', *IRB: A Review of Human Subjects Research*, 14:8 (1992) pp. 8-9.

3   For a fuller account of this development see the instructional videotape *Evolving Concern: Protection for Human Subjects* prepared by the National Institutes of Health and the Food and Drug Administration with the cooperation of the National Library of Medicine, U.S.A., to which we are indebted in this brief section.

4   Medical Research Council, 'Responsibilities in investigations on human subjects' in *Report of the Medical Research Council for the Year 1962-63*, London: H.M.S.O. (1964) pp. 21-5.

5   The World Medical Association. *The Declaration of Helsinki*. Recommendations guiding medical doctors in biomedical research involving human subjects. 1964 (Revised 1975 and 1983).

6   Department of Health and Social Security. *Supervision of the Ethics of Clinical Research Investigations and Fetal Research*, HSC(IS)153, London: D.H.S.S. (1975).

7   See Nicholson, R.H. (ed), *Medical Research with Children: Ethics, Law and Practice*, Oxford: Oxford University Press (1986), p. 4 & Chapter 8.

8   Department of Health, *Local Research Ethics Committees*, London: Department of Health (1991).

9   See, for example, Byrne, P., 'Medical research and the human subject: problems of consent and control in the UK experience', *Annals of the New York Academy of Science*, 530:144 (1988) and Neuberger, J., *Ethics and Health Care: the Role of Research Ethics Committees in the United Kingdom*, London: King's Fund Institute (1992), p. 45.

10 The two leading classical exponents of Utilitarianism, Jeremy Bentham and John Stuart Mill, were both philosophers and prominent social reformers. See Bentham, J., *An Introduction to the Principles of Morals and Legislation*, ed. J.H.Burns and H.L.A.Hart, London: Athlone Press (1970);   and Mill, J.S., 'Utilitarianism' in *Mill: Utilitarianism and Other Writings*, ed. M. Warnock, Glasgow: Collins (1962).

11 British Paediatric Association, *Guidelines for the Ethical Conduct of Medical Research Involving Children*, London: British Paediatric Association (1992), p. 4.

12 *op. cit.*, especially Chapters 3, 5 and 7.

13 See for instance the discussion of this and other revisions of utilitarianism in Griffin, J., *Well-being*, Oxford: Clarendon Press (1986), especially Part Two on 'Measurement'.

14 For instance, Hare, R.M., *Moral Thinking*, Oxford: Clarendon Press (1981), especially Chapters 5, 6 and 7.

15 See for instance Pellegrino, E. and Thomasma, D., *The Virtues in Medical Practice*, New York & Oxford: Oxford University Press (1993).

Chapter Two

The main job:
protecting the interests
of the research subject

2.1   Conflicting interests in clinical research

Damn it all, you can't have the crown of
thorns and *the thirty pieces of silver.*
(Aneurin Bevan)

A surprisingly large number of different interests are at stake in clinical
research.   Some of them are obvious, some less so;   equally, we can see quite
readily that some of the different interests are potentially in conflict with each
other, but some further potential conflicts of interest become apparent only on
closer inspection.   The most obvious interests are those of: **future patients**,
who need improved or entirely new therapies; **present patients** (many of whom
will also be among the future patients), who need at least the hope of such
improvements; **clinicians**, who need to be able to offer these same improved or
novel therapies to their patients, now and in the future;   and last but
demonstrably not least, the **research subject** (whether patient or healthy
volunteer), who needs assurances that any harms liable to arise in the research
will be minimised, and who in the case of patient volunteers needs also to be
confident that the possibilities of clinical benefit will not be significantly less
than those of the standard clinical management they would otherwise have
received.   The arguably less obvious interests include those of the **purchasers** of
health care, who need more cost-effective therapies (which will frequently,
though not necessarily, include therapies which are more effective in

straightforwardly clinical terms); the **sponsors of the research** who, if they are commercial companies such as the manufacturers of drugs or surgical equipment or appliances, need new markets, or a better share of existing markets; the **host research institution**, which needs the benefits of a continuing record of proven research achievements; and the **individual researcher**, who needs these same benefits in career terms. We should not overlook either the interests of patients' and research subjects' **close families, friends, guardians or dependants**. These latter interests are particularly apparent in the case of some especially vulnerable groups of patients who for a variety of reasons are unable to give consent on their own behalf to take part in research; in such cases the interests of parents or guardians come naturally into prominence, but it does not take much imagination to see that anyone who has an interest in the clinical recovery of a close relative or friend also has an interest in the decision as to whether their sick relative or friend should take part in relevant research.

Two things stand out from this list. The first is that conflicts of interest are not merely possible but pretty well inevitable. We all want medical research to be done; and generally speaking we all want it to be done on someone else. Since the above list includes the interests of research subjects, standard patients, researchers and sponsors among others, then this most obvious of conflicts is present many times over among the interests we have described. The second thing to stand out follows straightforwardly from the first. If conflicts of interest arise, then they have to be resolved, and the only practical means to this is to put the different kinds of interests in what we might call an order of moral priority: if we cannot simultaneously satisfy all interests, whose should we be most concerned to protect?

We shall take it for granted in this book that the simple and unequivocal answer to this question is: the interests of the research subject. This view is so widely accepted in modern Western medical practice, so well grounded in modern Western liberal thought, and moreover so firmly established at the heart of the whole institution of ethical review of clinical research, that we shall state it here without further justification, and we shall assume its truth in all of what follows. That is not to say that nothing further could be said in its support; indeed much of what we shall have to say will, we hope, draw attention to reasons for giving first place to the interests of the research subject. Neither is it to deny that a case can be made for an alternative view of moral priorities: after all, the utilitarian tradition, which we briefly surveyed in section 1.2, typically puts the general interests of the much larger numbers of present and future patients in first place. But our discussion of the present relation between the ideas of individual responsibilities and social responsibilities (section 1.3) nevertheless led us to the view that there were some individual sacrifices that society ought not to compel or to require. This in turn revealed the clinical research subject as a vulnerable

volunteer: and we recognised that to accept such a description is in itself to give ourselves morally compelling reasons for protecting the interests of the research subject first and foremost.

2.2 The special vulnerability of the research subject

I read the Book of Job last night. I don't think God comes well out of it.
(attributed to Virginia Woolf)

Clinical research subjects fall into either of two categories, normally sharply distinct.   Subjects are either patients themselves, on whom drugs and other treatments can be tested for their therapeutic effects as well as for any side effects, or they are healthy volunteers, on whom special comparisons can be made in order to isolate those effects in which researchers are interested. Patients need treatment anyway, so administering treatments to them under test conditions has an obvious clinical rationale;   the same is not true, however, of healthy volunteers and their participation can be justified only under special conditions which we shall examine particularly in sections 3.11 and 6.4.

The vulnerability of patients is obvious. People who are ill have a strong stake in getting better, and thus in cooperating with anyone they see as being in a position to help them get better. Clinicians also tend to be regarded socially as figures of authority; patients often defer towards, and express a sense of gratitude and obligation to, their doctors. It is easy for this deference to be abused, however unintentionally. And as we'll see, severely ill patients may have their decision-making faculties compromised by their illness, or they might retain these facilities yet still feel desperate to try anything that might help them get better. (Within the population of patients there are further sub-groups who are more than usually vulnerable, and we'll look more closely at them in sections 6.6 and 6.7.)

In one sense the vulnerability of healthy volunteers is less obvious; they aren't ill, and they enter the clinical context by choice, unlike most patients. But on further reflection, we must wonder what it is that makes some people choose to do something that most of us would far rather not do. And as we'll see later, the answer is all too frequently one of economic necessity, whereby the unemployed and those living in depressed areas provide the main source of volunteers when new drugs are to be injected into human beings for the first time. If anything constitutes vulnerability, economic hardship does. Something similiar is true of other groups who, traditionally, find it more than usually difficult to refuse invitations to volunteer: students, especially medical students, prisoners, members of the armed services, employees of pharmaceutical companies.   These groups' common characteristic is that of being in a position where it is not easy to refuse to do something which people would ordinarily significantly prefer not to do.

Once they have enrolled within a research project, the subjects' vulnerability becomes institutionalised. Their clinical management is now dictated by the needs of a scientific protocol as well as by their own physical condition. They may have a sense of obligation towards the researcher and towards their other clinical carers, making the subjects' later withdrawal from the research seem, if anything, more difficult than declining to take part in the first place. Subjects who are also patients might feel that their clinical interests will be compromised if they don't adhere strictly to the research regime, or to amendments to it which are subsequently proposed, however much they had been reassured to the contrary before enrolling. The general characteristics of an imbalance in power and knowledge as between clinician and patient are, if anything, intensified in the relation between clinical researcher and patient-subject; the aura and mystique of research contributes to this. The sense of making a socially useful contribution may propel someone into research in the first place – but it may then also seem to confine them there despite their feeling that they wished they were somewhere else.

This special vulnerability of all clinical research subjects is the moral springboard for the REC's concerns and responsibilities.

2.3   Putting limits on the price of benefits

'It is hard to be brave,' said Piglet, sniffing slightly,
'when you're only a Very Small Animal.'
(A.A. Milne)

Imagine a proposal to carry out the following research: a new drug is thought to offer a real hope of improved control of moderate to severe major depression in that proportion of patients who fail to respond to existing drugs. Preliminary studies on admittedly very small numbers of patients lead us to hope for better long-term outcome and for fewer side effects than is the case with the best currently available therapies. Major depressive illness, particularly in its moderate or severe forms, is a widespread and disabling condition which produces great suffering and, owing to the associated significantly increased risk of suicide, is potentially fatal. Patients whose illness is not well controlled by the existing drugs have much to gain from the introduction of a more effective drug. To find out whether the suspected improvement is real and reliable, a controlled test is necessary to compare the new drug with the best standard therapy. The test will work like this.

Equal numbers of comparably ill patients will be put into two groups, one to receive the current medication and the other to receive the new medication, and for four months these groups will be studied carefully for their progress, which will be analysed according to accepted techniques of assessment. Although the desired improvement may be a significant one, this can't yet be known; so to make the test sufficiently sensitive to detect a relatively small improvement, large numbers of patients need to be recruited into the research. To guard against bias creeping into the way that patients' progress is reported and recorded, the patients will be allocated between the groups at random, in such a way that neither they nor the researchers will know which drug any given patient is receiving during the trial period. Moreover, because we suspect that the new drug may interact with existing anti-depressant medications in unpredictable or harmful ways, patients who are to be given the trial drug cannot simply be transferred from current to new medication without a two-week long 'washout' period – during which no medication must be taken. And, obviously, to preserve the patients' and researchers' ignorance concerning which treatment anyone is actually getting, both the group receiving the new drug and the group receiving the current drug must be treated alike, and both must undergo this 'washout' period. Finally, since the whole necessity of this research project lies in the fact that we only suspect and do **not** know for certain whether the new drug is really any better than the old one, there is no guarantee that across larger numbers of patients the drug will prove effective at all. The proposed study is meant to confirm whether earlier suspicions of a benefit, based on preliminary studies in very small numbers of patients, are correct.

If we add all this together, we see that the proposed research will be capable of identifying and confirming perhaps small but nonetheless important improvements in the clinical management of a very serious condition, **or** of confirming current standard medication as being the best available; without doing the research we will lack the information clinicians need to be confident that they are prescribing the best available drug for this condition. Either way, the benefits of the research seem compelling. These benefits will moreover be enjoyed by society at large, in terms of the other present and future sufferers of major depressive illness, sufferers who are playing no part in the present trial.

But when we add together all the features of the trial we will recognise also that it involves taking large numbers of patients with a serious and potentially life-threatening condition and withdrawing them entirely from active treatment for a two-week period. Following that period we will be placing half of them on an unproven treatment of unknown efficacy for a further four months. Withdrawn from treatment, their condition can deteriorate unpredictably, and in some cases perhaps fatally. Now it seems that the price of the research may be considerable. Moreover, and unlike the benefits of the research, the price is essentially paid by the individual patients actually taking part in it. In trying to decide whether the research should go ahead, we are inevitably asking whether the benefits can justify the price that might be paid. And in asking that, we are also implicitly asking whether there is any amount of benefit that could ever justify the very highest price that we can foresee.

This piece of proposed research presents us with a difficult moral judgement precisely because it lies in an indeterminate area between clear extremes. Some clinical research carries essentially low risks; for instance the comparative evaluation of topical cream applications for minor inflammatory skin conditions involves no obvious significant harms to the research subjects, provided that they are taking part voluntarily, that they have been carefully recruited according to strict entry criteria, and that the research is well designed and well conducted. Assuming that there were reason to hope that one among the creams being compared might emerge as even marginally more useful than the others (and no reason to think any of the creams was ineffective or poorly tolerated), it is hard to see why anyone would find this research morally troubling. At the other extreme is research whose risks are so overwhelming that virtually no one would even consider carrying it out. It is, fortunately, easier to find historical rather than contemporary examples of this kind of research: one of the grossest (and certainly most widely reported) examples concerned the deliberate infection of mentally retarded but physically healthy children in Willowbrook State School, New York, with viral hepatitis, extracted from the faeces of infected children and administered orally[1]. Even were there to be real and scientifically respectable benefits from research of this sort, and even were it to be conducted on willing adult volunteers rather than on what were, effectively, child prisoners, it is hard to think that any Research Ethics Committee would allow a proposal for such research to proceed. In rejecting it, they would be judging a certain risk of harm as **intrinsically** unacceptable, incapable of being justified morally no matter what plausible benefits were claimed from the research.

Just by virtue of being so clear, these two extremes give us no real difficulties in deciding how we should judge them. The difficulty with the controlled trial of the new anti-depressant medication is just that it is really not like either of these extreme cases. Neither the condition of major depression, nor the inevitably potent and somewhat unpredictable medication used to combat it, is trivial or innocuous like irritable skin or topical skin cream. On the other hand the risks of the trial, including those of the 'washout' period, might be at least arguably commensurate with these patients' need for better (or better tolerated) control of their distressing and disabling condition – unlike the wholly new and gratuitous risk of grave illness or death which was cynically imposed on the under-nourished but nevertheless essentially non-diseased New York orphans. So the questions facing us are therefore these: given that certain risks could never justifiably be imposed upon clinical research subjects, but given also that we think it acceptable for volunteers to face finite, minor harms in pursuit of the benefits which clinical research could provide, where do we draw the line? How shall we decide where to draw it? And how shall we police the line once it is drawn?

In the first section of this chapter we identified the overriding task of the Research Ethics Committee as being that of protecting the research subject's interests. Next we confirmed that task in the light of the research subject's special vulnerability. Now we have begun to locate that overriding task in a recognition of the price that must be paid for the benefits which clinical research can bring us. The detailed working-out of this overriding task and of its practical implications will form the subject matter of the rest of this book.

Notes

1   Nicholson, R., *Medical Research with Children*, Oxford: Oxford University Press (1986), pp. 29-30.

Chapter Three

Research design and methodology: built-in risks

Perfection of planned layout is achieved only by institutions on the point of collapse.
(C. Northcote Parkinson)

3.1   Varieties of research on human subjects

It is incident to physicians, I am afraid, beyond all other
men, to mistake subsequence for consequence.
(Samuel Johnson)

There is a large variety of kinds of research carried out on human subjects
which it is the responsibility of Research Ethics Committees to review. Some of
these do not involve 'bedside contacts' with the research subjects and may not
strictly be called clinical studies. However the studies RECs should be
responsible for are those where the well-being of the subject is in any way
possibly threatened by the research. Thus it will still be the REC's
responsibility to monitor certain examples of research which is not strictly
concerned with health issues – for example some psychological research such as
an examination of the relation between alcohol consumption and aggression –
since the stresses or stimuli to which the research subject is subjected or the
induced states and resulting measurement to which that person may be subjected
could be detrimental to his well-being. By and large, however, the vast majority
of the research which is presented to RECs is clinical research in the narrow
sense, though it may range much wider than medicine into nursing,
physiotherapy, surgery and other health care specialisms involving patient
contact, and indeed into management studies. The main categories of research
coming before the REC are these:

(a) Pharmaceutical studies

Most protocols presented to the REC for review will concern the development and/or the use of pharmaceutical products. Such research is divided into distinct phases, both to protect the research subjects and, connectedly, to concentrate in the correct order on different aspects of the properties of new medicines. We will say more about each of these phases in section 3.2.

(b) Other therapeutic regime studies

Many clinical trials are designed to compare and evaluate treatment regimes which are not centrally based on the development of drugs. For example, it may be of interest to researchers to compare the outcomes of day-surgery patients with hospitalised patients for a given indication, or to compare the effects of delayed clamping of the umbilical cord in pre-term neonates with the standard practice, or to compare giving patients anti-emetics before their anaesthetic with giving them the same preparations after surgery, in the recovery room.

(c) Trials of new or modified technologies

Sometimes new technologies are developed in the hope that they will mark an improvement on the current tools available to health care professionals. Before these tools can be compared they must first be tested to see whether they offer a real chance of improvements. This may involve their application on small numbers of cases, very carefully monitored. For example, the authors once reviewed a trial in which a new, non-invasive technology for measuring heart function in the developing foetus was to be tested on a small group of pregnant women[1], and on another occasion reviewed a trial to explore the idea that the direction in which a spinal anaesthetic injection was orientated in the patient influenced the amount of anaesthetic effect produced.

(d) Epidemiological studies

These studies usually involve professionals who do not have responsibility for the care of the patients to be studied; they often need to access details of the medical records of patients in order to collate, for example, the incidences of disease conditions, the outcomes of various treatment measures, demographic indicators, population trends and so on. There are special issues attaching to review of research of this kind and we will consider them more fully in section 3.8. This sort of research does not involve trials as such, but it does require the collection and analysis of health data which may itself produce, amongst other things, new hypotheses to be tested in subsequent clinical trials with respect to the causes of disease and ill-health.

(e) Public health surveys

These studies are closer to epidemiological studies than to clinical trials. They too involve accessing demographic health data. They are essentially concerned with the control of disease and the protection of public health. Examples of such research would be the conducting of National Risk Surveys or prevalence studies charting the extent and incidence of specific (frequently infectious) diseases. The chief difference between these studies and epidemiological studies is that the public health surveys include the collection of data from actual sufferers or relations of sufferers and therefore they present different issues for consideration by RECs.

(f) Psychological and other behavioural research

We have already pointed out that psychological research might not always entail researching into issues of health. Nevertheless the potential impact of such research on the health of research subjects makes the ethical review of psychological research protocols a proper part of the business of RECs. Of course psychological research is often specifically concerned with health issues. An example would be the quantitative study of the responses of individuals and groups of people to various kinds of stress, or the testing of a new therapeutic intervention involving behaviour modification.

Some psychological and behavioural research involves what are known as 'qualitative research' methodologies that are frequently ill-understood and ill-appreciated by REC members who more typically have been trained in quantitative scientific techniques. Many nursing research projects fall within the broad category of behavioural studies and use qualitative methodologies; a typical example might be the study of the long-term effects of bereavement on the widows of deceased Alzheimer's disease patients, by means of extended or serial interviews with the research subjects. (In our experience such proposals are not always well served by being presented in the language of philosophical phenomenology, of which relatively few of the applicants in question seem able to give a convincing account.)

(g) Other cases

There are other studies which fall across the boundaries between clinical practice, management and research. The sorts of cases that might fall under this description are various examples of clinical practice (such as the Munchausen syndrome by proxy case discussed in section 4.4), patient satisfaction surveys, clinical audits and staff studies (such as the study of the levels of stress suffered by nurses on an intensive care unit). It might be difficult in some cases to determine whether such studies should be subjected to ethical review or not. However, in the United Kingdom the Department of Health has issued some very sensible advice on this matter, which it is worth quoting at length:

> On the face of it, all 'research proposals' involving NHS patients or access to NHS premises must go before the LREC. However when the [advice] on LRECs was drawn up, ... it was never intended that it should apply to the sort of surveys [described]. These are important for management and monitoring purposes, and should not as a rule raise ethical issues.
>
> But on the other hand there is an important principle here – namely that it should not be left to researchers themselves to decide whether their research poses ethical issues, and hence whether to seek LREC clearance. Even 'customer satisfaction' surveys about hospital food or signposting might stray into ethical areas if approaches were made to, say, terminally ill people or the recently bereaved.
>
> We therefore take the view that, although non-medical surveys would not normally be expected to go before the LREC, those carrying out such a survey should nevertheless send details to the LREC Chairman. The Chairman should be able to confirm that the survey can go ahead without having to put it to the full LREC.[2]

3.2   The phases of drug development

It was my uncle who discovered that alcohol was food well in advance of medical thought.
(P.G. Wodehouse)

There are four phases in the clinical development of new medicines. They are preceded by intensive and prolonged preclinical trials involving animal studies. Ethical review procedures concern the clinical development phases; these all involve the use of human subjects. (Figure 1 at the end of this chapter provides a useful overview of the phases of drug development, their timescales, subject numbers, costs and attrition rates[3].)

3.2.1 Phase I studies

These studies involve the use of healthy volunteer subjects (whose special circumstances are considered in more detail in section 3.11). After prolonged testing on animals to establish a drug's general actions and its safety in principle, Phase I research administers the new drug to humans for the first time.

The research subjects in this phase are almost always healthy volunteers, though there are some exceptions such as where cytotoxic (anti-cancer) drugs are to be tested. The main reason why these exceptional substances should not be tested initially on healthy subjects is that they are necessarily very toxic, and the risk of serious adverse events is unacceptably high. There are still ethical problems involved in testing them on seriously ill patients, who are the only subject group which can defensibly be used for such testing, because their circumstances make consent a more difficult matter. But given that such patients are *in extremis* and that the trial substance might hold out some slender hope of palliating their symptoms or slowing the progress of their disease, the balance between risk and benefit to the subject is totally different from that involving healthy volunteers. (The problems of weighing risks and benefits and of being confident about the value of specific consents are explored in Chapters Five and Six.) Generally the first-time application of such substances occurs in the context of 'last ditch' clinical practice rather than in a formal clinical trial setting.

At Phase I it is most important to discover what constitutes a safe dose of the substance, as well as how that substance is absorbed, whether adequate amounts of it are to be found in the blood, how fast the substance is eliminated from the body, what concentrations of the substance can be delivered to relevant parts of the body and so on. After safety, these **pharmacokinetics** are the main focus of interest, though additionally the drug's **pharmacodynamic** effects (or actions) may be detected at Phase I; any unwanted effects, if serious, would themselves place question marks over the drug's usefulness. At the same time, other effects such as lowering of blood pressure might suggest additional useful applications for the drug. Because many substances such as antibiotic medicines are not meant to produce effects in healthy subjects, beneficial effects are not generally the research target in this phase of investigation.

3.2.2   Phase II studies[4]

At Phase II researchers are concerned more with the possible efficacy of a substance and with establishing the related useful dosages. Clearly all research subjects in this phase have to be patients suffering from the condition(s) the drug is meant to help. But safety and tolerability are still important: this phase involves repeated dosings, and the healthy and the sick might metabolise the drug differently, revealing new dangers. Additionally, the range of subjects may be wider at this phase in terms of gender and age, although their total numbers should still be quite restricted (see Figure 1, p. 50). The researchers best fitted for this phase of clinical development are those especially familiar with the disease conditions for which the new medicine is being developed.

3.2.3   Phase III studies

The only drugs entering Phase III are those which at Phase II looked therapeutically promising and were well tolerated by research subjects. This is the final phase before the marketing of a drug; researchers try to establish definitively the drug's safety and efficacy (degree of benefit) by testing it on much larger numbers of patients for much longer periods. By the end of this phase researchers must be able to state clearly all the indications for which the drug is to be used and specify precisely what dosages, methods of administration and contraindications of the drug apply. If this phase is satisfactorily completed manufacturers may apply for a product licence.

3.2.4   Phase IV studies

This final, follow-up, phase involves still larger numbers of patient treatments over a much longer period than the Phase III studies. The drug is now formally prescribed as an effective medicine. However researchers still need to study its long-term beneficial and harmful effects, to compare its usefulness with that of other relevant drugs, to identify any interactions with other drugs patients might be taking concurrently, to see whether there are better dosage levels and of course to pick out other possible uses. In reviewing this phase of research we must try to pick out serious follow-up work from mere marketing ploys – not always an easy matter.

3.3   Study aims and the null hypothesis

*The music teacher came twice each week to bridge
the awful gap between Dorothy and Chopin.*
(George Ade)

The essence of research concerns resolving uncertainty – typically in the context of medical research, uncertainty about the bio-availability, benefits and safety of existing and envisaged therapies. The uncertainty frequently concerns, not so much whether a particular therapy is any good at all, as how well it compares with existing therapies of (approximately) known value. If research aims at resolving uncertainty then research is redundant unless that uncertainty is really there in the first place; what's more, given that performing the research involves finite risks to individuals and as such has some moral cost, then it is unethical to perform research that is redundant. It follows from this that for research to be ethically sound, there must be some degree of genuine uncertainty about the value of the therapy being investigated.

Characteristically, research is designed to show the truth or otherwise of a particular proposition, itself constructed to express the uncertainty in question. If we are uncertain whether or not new drug B is more effective than existing drug A, we might express this by devising a proposition, 'Drug B is better than drug A' and then testing it for its truth. However, how much better must the drug be for the proposition to be true? To have a testable proposition we would have to specify in advance the extent of the hypothetical advantage, and this seems difficult and obscure. Assuming some sort of measuring scale on which benefits could be measured (itself a problem, discussed in Chapter Five) then the trouble with arbitrarily proposing a 10% improvement, and discovering only an 8% improvement, is that it leads to the somewhat misleading falsification of the study hypothesis.

What we are really interested in is whether there is any extra benefit in the new drug, and if so, in how big that increment turns out to be. The best way of addressing this is to test the proposition that there is no difference at all between drug A and drug B. The proposition will be falsified by any positive or negative difference; moreover the proposition is easy to specify and it is straightforward to conceptualise. This proposition is the conventional way of expressing what is therefore called the null hypothesis. Typical clinical research aims at testing the relevant null hypothesis for the therapy in which we are interested.

This approach can be maintained even when there is no existing standard therapy as a comparator, such as in the treatment of Alzheimer's Disease. In this case the comparator can be a supposedly inactive substance or placebo. Placebos pose important and interesting problems of their own and are discussed in section

3.6; however it is reasonable to suppose that if there is presently no known active or effective treatment, and we do not know whether the proposed new treatment is active or effective, then the null hypothesis which we should test is that there is no difference in effectiveness between the proposed new treatment and placebo.

One of the problems with establishing a null hypothesis concerns its obvious artificiality: there is no guarantee, and often no likelihood, that the researcher either believes it or even has an open mind on it. A researcher may be convinced that the new treatment offers some advantage over existing therapies, but may lack hard evidence and may be uncertain as to whether the advantage is significant. Ideally the research ought to test a hypothesis which adequately captures genuine uncertainty genuinely held by the researcher – the more so since we have specified that some genuine uncertainty is a necessary condition of ethically proper research. Thus, if a null hypothesis could be identified which properly expressed the researcher's actual uncertainty, that would be better than one which did not. However, the arbitrariness of specifying degrees of advantage, and the difficulties of testing them as compared to the testing of zero advantage or 'therapeutic equipoise', provide good practical reasons for the conventional null hypothesis. The moral requirement of genuine uncertainty therefore applies more importantly to the overall, general knowledge and beliefs of the researcher (and proposer and sponsor) than to the precise conventional form in which the uncertainty is expressed for the purposes of the trial. Nevertheless it is obviously vital that the research be capable of testing the null hypothesis, and furthermore of doing so in a way that will genuinely cast light on the actual uncertainty which is at stake.

3.4 Multiple objectives and scientific validity

Well, if I called the wrong number, why did you answer the phone?
(James Thurber)

There are both good scientific reasons and strong practical reasons for ensuring that a study has clear and focused **objectives**. There should preferably be only one of these and certainly not more than three. They should be reflected in the small number of **endpoints** of the study, and one of these should be selected as definitive. These objectives and endpoints must determine the study design, and should be followed through by the study's statistical plan. Any interesting results outside these strictly defined endpoints should be regarded only as an exercise in generating hypotheses rather than as proper testing; they should not be claimed as 'positive results'[5].

3.4.1   The temptation to multiply objectives

Given that the aim in clinical research is to obtain answers to therapeutically important questions, and given that the benefits of doing so are bought at a price, then we might feel morally compelled to get as many answers as possible from a given piece of research using a given number of research subjects. In this way the moral 'unit price' of research benefits would seem to be kept low. Unfortunately this manoeuvre will rarely work, because the methodological penalties for trying simultaneously to answer multiple questions are serious. Suppose we came across a study on healing leg ulcers that included as its objectives establishing claims about:

- clinically relevant healing;
- reduction in ulcer size;
- reduction in amputation rate;
- alleviation of ischaemic pain;
- reduction in analgesic consumption;
- safety;
- tolerability;
- quality of life.

These multiple objectives betray a failure by the researcher to define precisely what he or she is trying to do. It is a 'scattergun' approach which does no more than list the unpleasant consequences of the disease in the hope that at least one of them may be helped by the intervention under examination. Some of the objectives share the same variables – for example, we might ask whether it is necessary to include both pain reduction and reduced analgesic consumption, or again, both healing of the ulcer and reduction of size. In fact in both cases the duplication of objective is simply a duplication of the method of measurement. There is no clear idea of what the experiment is likely to achieve or of what is important to the patient. Sometimes such unclarity is disguised by the generalisation of objectives such as 'to compare the safety and tolerability of treatment A with treatment B'.

These features invite scientific, ethical and practical criticisms of such studies, and it is worth our while considering each of these kinds of criticism in turn.

3.4.2   Scientific criticism of multiple objectives

There are two main purposes of a scientific experiment: to generate new hypotheses and to test a specific hypothesis. Most medical experiments are of the second type, although they may result in new hypotheses generated as a 'spin-off' from incidental observations in the course of the experiment. An experiment to test a specific hypothesis in strict laboratory conditions should therefore have a single objective marked out by a strictly limited range of endpoints. Multiple or ill-defined objectives leave open the choice of endpoints of the study. Although it may appear that tightly drafted statistical procedures with properly defined endpoints offer some compensation for ill-defined objectives, in reality the objectives are meaningless, an exercise in box filling.

Without tight statistical control of the validity and significance of data, the researcher may finish a study with ten or more possible endpoints to choose from. In an asthma study there might be lung function tests at 30 minutes and 60 minutes, peak flow at the same intervals, peak flow measured at home, blood oxygen and carbon dioxide levels, use of relief medication, diary card records, physician's global assessment and so forth. If any of these is shown to be favourable this can subsequently be claimed as the chosen endpoint and the study declared to be a success.

Where statistical significance **is** properly indicated, the results may not be sufficient for realising the objective of a study. For example, even where a difference between two treatments is shown to be statistically significant, more work may be required to establish a positive conclusion – it depends on the degree of difference regarded as **clinically** significant for the condition or treatment in question. The normal level of statistical significance is that there be no more than one chance in twenty that a given result is due to random variation - an average of no more than one out of twenty results analysed should be a misleading 'false positive'. If the parameters of clinical significance are not specified, then clearly the more results there are to analyse the greater the chance that a researcher will appear to strike lucky regardless of the true effect of the treatment: even if no positive result on the question of efficacy is forthcoming from a study, it may still be tempting to search for some return on the side of safety, such as a difference in blood chemistry or haematology. Whilst 'data dredging' of this kind might be difficult to get away with in a pharmaceutical company trial where regulatory authorities provide experienced and critical evaluators of data, there are real possibilities in less strict contexts of such results appearing as 'publishable'.

3.4.3   Ethical criticism of multiple objectives

It is important to note that poor science in research involving human subjects is inherently unethical in that it subjects people to discomfort, inconvenience and possibly risk for no good purpose.   The kind of approach referred to above in the ulcer treatment example is tantamount to the researcher saying 'I'm going to give this treatment to these patients and see what happens'.   But is this a sufficiently rigorous approach to justify putting ill, elderly, distressed patients through an ordeal by measurement (such as endoscopic examination) and to the risk of toxicity?

The fact is that multiple objectives give a licence for multiple investigations. Most people have a sense of privacy about their bodies. The amount of touching and intimate manipulation that most of us permit even to close friends and relations is strictly limited.   Should we not respect that sense that humans normally feel for their bodies as a defended area?   In addition there are the demands upon endurance produced by long and often poorly organised investigation.   Patients are, almost by definition, in less than perfect health, many are very ill indeed and many are old.   It is not unusual for a study to involve quite tiring procedures such as treadmill exercises, or lung function tests, to which may be added a chest X-ray, a visit to an ECG facility, a visit to the laboratory and finally to the pharmacy to collect medication.   It should not be forgotten that many investigations carry a risk. The Royal College of Radiologists, for instance, have called attention to the risks even of simple chest X-rays. Every time a new objective is added to a study there is a good chance that a new investigation will be added, whereas if objectives were clearly focused a number of investigations would be seen for what they are: in the 'while we're at it' class.

3.4.4   Practical criticism of multiple objectives

It is a general experience that the more data collected, the poorer their quality.   This may be because of simple physical limitations.   In a pharmacokinetic study, for example, there may be timed blood samples at perhaps ten-minute intervals.   There may be a number of subjects being processed simultaneously. The fact that there is an intravenous cannula in place does not greatly increase the speed of collection, since not only must blood be withdrawn but also the cannula must be flushed with heparin, there may be multiple blood samples to be placed in different anticoagulants and tubes must be labelled and racked. If to this is added the measuring of blood pressure, ECG, respiratory rate and oral temperature, it may simply be impossible to perform this in the time available. This can be detrimental to the study if samples are contaminated with heparin or mislabelled – but it can be dangerous or even lethal to the patient if, owing to haste, there is cross-contamination between patients. For disaster to occur there need be only one HIV carrier in the group.

Even where data is collected in a more leisurely environment, over-investigation means long sessions with loss of concentration by researchers or fatigue in patients, both of which can lead to poor or misleading data. For instance, how many psychometric tests can be performed in one day and still produce valid results? Properly focused objectives lead to relevant data of good quality rather than to a mix of relevant and irrelevant data, abundant but of indifferent quality.

3.5   Scientific rigour and the problem of controls

My face is the same and the scripts are the same; only the horses change.
(Audie Murphy, comparing his forty-odd appearances in cowboy films.)

Research aims at moving away from uncertainty towards something more like actual certainty: at any rate towards knowledge in which we can have the highest reasonable confidence. Moreover this confidence must be capable of being extended beyond the circumstances of the research itself: research is concerned with what happens to the patients or volunteers being studied, not for their own sakes but for the sake of what can be learned regarding other, future and as yet unknown patients. In other words, what is learned from the trial will be of limited usefulness unless it can be generalised beyond the trial.

An obstacle to this is the obvious variability of different individual patients: we need to be confident that the very different individual constitution and circumstances of Smith (whom we have never met) will not defy our hope that he will respond, to the therapy under investigation, in the same way as Jones (who is enrolled in our study now). That requires our being certain that Jones' response is due to factors which are common to different people in relevantly similar circumstances (having the same illness to the same degree, for instance) and not due to factors which are specific to Jones and unlikely to be found in Smith (such as Jones's food intolerances or other metabolic idiosyncrasies). We also need to be sure that Jones' response has nothing to do with the circumstances of the experiment itself: for instance, psychological expectations on his part or even on the part of the researcher herself, such as in cases where one or both of them know that great hopes rest on the innovative treatment being administered. Less obviously, we also need to be sure the apparent results don't stem from material complications, such as the additionally attentive nursing care that might be provided to the research subjects, special diets or other environmental factors in the facility concerned, or from the fact that Jones (or Smith) comes from a local ethnic cluster which is more susceptible, or for that matter more resistant, to certain diseases.

So for research to be capable of being generalised, it must screen out all those individual variables, leaving only the factors which can be presumed to apply to all relevantly similar cases. This is ordinarily done by the use of **controls**. Controls are other research subjects who are matched as closely as possible, in all respects except one, to the research subjects on whom the trial therapy is being tested. Thus, all the variables suggested above, concerning diet, style of care, ethnic background (but also age, sex and general physical condition where relevant) should be similarly present in both the primary study patients and the control patients. The one single respect in which they differ is the trial therapy itself: the patients in the primary study group receive it, and the patients in the control group do not. In this way, if there is a difference in therapeutic response so that those receiving active treatment do better than those not receiving it, it is highly probable that the improvement results from receiving the treatment, since this is the only significant difference between the circumstances of the two groups. If the only difference between the Smiths and the Joneses is that the Smiths get the treatment and the Joneses don't, then if the Smiths get better as well we can be pretty confident it's because they got the treatment.

The moral problem with all this is obvious: what happens if the Joneses need treatment as much as do the Smiths, but they don't get it? Obviously if the groups really **are** similar in all other relevant respects, the Joneses certainly **do** need treatment. So can we be justified in using patients, who need an active treatment, as controls? The answer to this is complex, and reflects the fact that there are different kinds of controls: in most of these kinds, the control group can and does receive an active treatment, typically the standard or best existing therapy. If the null hypothesis expresses or represents a genuine uncertainty as to whether the new therapy being studied is better than the current standard, then the control group indeed are receiving the best available treatment, so far as anybody knows. This in itself illustrates the moral importance of there being genuine uncertainty regarding the benefits of the trial therapy.

Other kinds of controls may be appropriate when a prospective comparison of active treatments in large groups of patients is not possible. These include using a particular patient as his 'own control', notably in chronic diseases, where each of two treatments being compared is given to the same patient over separate periods of time. In these studies the order in which treatments are given is usually chosen at random. (This approach also offers a variation on the prospective randomised controlled trial: in the 'crossover' trial, the trial therapy and the comparator therapy are switched half-way through the study period.) Historical controls compare current patients with other subjects who have previously been treated with a drug or other form of intervention, and for whom the results are already known.

Obviously patients who are suffering a significant illness and who do need continuing active treatment should not be denied active treatment through being entered into a trial: the kinds of controls employed should not as a matter of **design** exclude anyone who needs an active treatment from receiving it, although we must recognise that trial therapies may on occasion turn out to be less effective than the standard treatment or even inactive or harmful; in being entered into research a patient should understand the possibility of this happening and there should be clear procedures for responding to the needs of patients who are evidently not receiving effective treatment at a time when they need it. There are special problems in using children or other vulnerable subjects as controls; we will say more about this when we discuss these particular subject groups in Chapter Six.

Clearly the design of controlled studies necessarily involves a compromise between the demands of scientific rigour and the needs of those patients who are used as controls. Once the strict null hypothesis is reasonably doubted, we face a compelling reason to ensure that all patients who need the best active treatment actually get it. But reasonable doubt is not conclusive doubt, and the drive for certainty will sometimes have to be compromised in the protection of the patients' interests: we will have to settle for what is merely **probable**. The point at which this compromise must be reached – and the degree of probability that will be settled for – will vary with the seriousness of the relevant illness conditions and the margin of any supposed emerging therapeutic advantages. Research protocols should specify how these compromises will be reached (for instance, the study endpoints should be clear and appropriate for the disease in question) and leave REC members in no doubt that patients' interests will indeed be protected.

3.6 Randomisation and its implications

Every Tom, Dick and Harry is called Arthur.
(Sam Goldwyn)

The need for prior allocation of patients to the different groups within the trial intensifies the difficulties already examined in connection with the general problem of controls. As an integral part of the process of testing active responses against the responses from a matched control group, the researcher needs to be confident that no unconscious but influential criteria creep into the selection process which determines who goes into the control group and who into the active group. Clearly, for instance, people who are more acutely ill might show a more visibly dramatic response to an effective therapy than people who are more mildly ill; alternatively, people whose general mobility is slightly reduced may show a slower or reduced response to certain kinds of therapy (for instance, drugs to improve joint mobility might appear to 'do less for' patients whose activity is already restricted owing to shortness of breath). It is important that all such characteristics are either excluded altogether or, if not, then distributed equally between the active and the control groups, and not allowed to accumulate in the one or the other group as a result of the allocation choices of the researcher – consciously or unconsciously. In other words the researcher should not choose who goes into which group. The obvious way to avoid this is for the distribution among the groups to be done by (valid) randomisation.

Further, we noticed that researchers must try and prevent their own and their subjects' expectations and beliefs from influencing the research outcomes. If we believe we are getting something that will make us well, we will often get well on account simply of the belief, despite the fact that we are receiving nothing more than an inert preparation of lactose: unfortunately a proportion of the harmful side-effects of active drugs will also be mimicked in patients receiving placebo[6]. (The seemingly preposterous repertoire of the power of belief extends even to responses to the colour of pills, with red placebos being particularly effective in some circumstances[7].) By the same token, the researcher may 'see' the improvements she expects to see in patients whom she knows to be receiving active treatment, and miss or at any rate underestimate improvements in the control group. So it is important (where possible) that while the research is being conducted the researcher should not know which subjects are in which group, any more than she should choose which group they be allocated to in the first place. Equally the subjects should not know which group they are in either, in order that their expectations not interfere with their progress, actual, reported or observed. Thus the ideal study of this kind would be not merely randomised but also 'blind' or 'double-blind' in that neither patient nor researcher knows whether the patient is receiving an active therapy. In this way it is hoped that the individual variables in response can be minimised to the fullest degree possible. (Whether a trial actually can be made blind or double-blind will depend on whether the research therapy is one which can be made to resemble closely the existing standard therapy or placebo which is used for the control group(s). This is obviously an easier matter when testing drugs than when when testing surgical procedures or appliances.)

In general terms the main ethical problem with randomisation is that it severs the ordinary connection between the patient and the therapy chosen by his doctor as being most appropriate for him as an individual: the therapy is chosen not by the personal decision of the physician but by a mechanical procedure designed to avoid individual considerations, that is, a random decision procedure (albeit choosing from among alternatives that lie within clinically prudent limits).

The research patient gives up his usual clinical expectations of individually-tailored treatment on entering randomised controlled trials. The REC will want to be certain that this is appropriate for the kind of patient and the kind of illness condition concerned, and that the patient fully understands this on agreeing to enter the trial. (The general problem of ordinary treatment expectations is one considered in more detail in section 3.10.) This general problem is obviously intensified if the responsible clinicians do not even know what treatment the patient is receiving in the event of a double-blind trial. Here it is vital that, in the event of the patient becoming more ill than expected, or failing to make expected or clinically desired improvements, or in any other circumstance which gives cause for clinical concern, it can quickly be established what treatment the patient is in fact receiving so that steps can be taken to adjust his management. Obviously this means withdrawing him from the research: the REC will want to be satisfied that any proposed research incorporates prompt and effective measures to do this, including the prompt breaking of any codes involved in the randomisation process, and swift notification of the patient's doctor.

3.7   Patients, placebos and sub-optimal treatment

> *The Queen's powder-blue dress and tilted wide-brimmed*
> *hat made the garden party seem more real.*
> (The *Observer* newspaper, recalled by Susan Stebbings)

Is it morally permissible ever to give patients less than the best treatment? Precisely this is typically required by the idea of placebo-controlled trials and indeed by any controlled trial involving comparisons between different treatments of which only one has known therapeutic properties. The risk of giving patients less than the best is of course built into the idea of research anyway, since genuine research is, as we have seen, characterised by genuine uncertainty. But there seems a clear moral difference between saying, in the ordinary clinical care of an individual patient, 'I don't know whether or not this treatment will help you, but nothing else that we have tried has helped you so it is worth trying this' and saying, to a pool of patients who are prospective trial subjects, 'I don't know which of you will get an active treatment and which of you will get a dummy treatment, but I hope at the end of the trial that we'll see whether there is any difference between those of you who got the active treatment and those of you who got the dummy treatment'. The difference lies between the individual clinical encounter on the one hand, where there is of course often genuine uncertainty, but an uncertainty which must be addressed in the context always of matching the patient's needs with the best treatments known to the clinician, even where their effectiveness proves to be elusive; and the de-individualised research context on the other hand, where the uncertainty is a systematic one, and is in one sense designed-in by the researcher in the interests of advancing knowledge.

It seems clear then that the circumstances in which it is morally justifiable to put patients into a placebo-controlled trial are fairly strictly limited: (i) there must be a genuine uncertainty as to whether the proposed treatment is any more likely to help the patients concerned than is a placebo; (ii) in most cases there must be no agreed alternative treatment of greater therapeutic value than placebo. Exceptions to this could arise if the statistical advantage of using a 'coarse' comparator like placebo enable a much smaller trial to be run as a result, though such trials give a very poor picture of the rival merits of the active drugs themselves and as such may be of doubtful value; (iii) there must be a significant need for the knowledge to be obtained by the placebo-controlled trial (it must be an important question whether the proposed treatment is better than placebo); (iv) there must be a reasonable possibility that the proposed new treatment can indeed turn out to be better than placebo. We can see at once that it is not entirely easy to fulfil both condition (i) and condition (iv), though it is certainly possible; generally this will happen when the treatment under investigation has what is envisaged as being the right sort of chemical or molecular basis to be active (perhaps, typically, when seen in the light of novel discoveries in our understanding of the way the body works) **and** is also the first of its type to be tried. Placebo-controlled trials should be the exception and not the norm, and it should take exceptional circumstances to justify them.

To these four conditions we might add: (v) the illness from which the patients are suffering must not be so serious that any delay in their receiving an active treatment would be clinically harmful or dangerous. In this case, even when there is genuine uncertainty as to whether the proposed treatment will offer any advantage over placebo, seriously ill patients must receive whatever treatment is actually available or, when no demonstrated treatment is available, there is a good case for thinking that they should be offered the proposed new treatment. We might say that the patient should receive the benefit of the doubt, even when the doubt concerns the proposed new treatment. In effect, of course, this means that seriously ill patients and rigorously-controlled research usually do not mix: research should normally be put aside in favour of experimental clinical treatment, where the only control or comparator is the patient himself.

The REC will want to be satisfied, then, that all the above conditions are met when research is proposed that includes a placebo comparator group. Much the same kinds of considerations (with the obvious exception of condition (ii)) apply to ordinary control groups using standard available treatments: the difference lies in the fact that here the conditions are much more readily met. Condition (v) applies a little less straightforwardly though it is still importantly true. Whether in fact a given research subject will have received the treatment best for him in the course of a randomised controlled trial will remain unknown, unless the trial is of a crossover design such that all subjects will at different times in the trial find themselves in both the comparator arms (and even here other factors may be at work in the clinical progress of any given patient). However, the seriously ill patient needs whatever his doctor thinks best for him, and his treatment should be randomised only in the circumstance of absolute uncertainty about which option is best. This circumstance is likely to be rare except in the case where both (a) there is simply no current effective treatment and (b) the proposed new treatment offers only a hypothetical, and not a probable, advantage. Lastly the REC should be highly sceptical of any double-blind randomised trials involving seriously ill patients; the justification for not **choosing** into which group the seriously ill patient is put cannot usually extend to a justification for not **knowing** into which group that patient has been put. Rapid adjustments to the patient's management, more necessary with the seriously ill and most necessary of all with the acutely ill, will usually require the doctor to know what treatment the patient is receiving from first to last.

3.8   Epidemiological research

Red-haired people are poor at history.
(Anonymous Oxford history examiner)

The characteristics of epidemiological research are that it involves collecting and analysing information about very large numbers of patients, whose individual identities are generally unimportant, and that it typically involves doing so outside the clinical setting. Epidemiologists are typically concerned with the incidence and prevalence of disease conditions, with the environmental and social factors associated with specific disease conditions and perhaps causing them, and with the implications of knowledge of this kind for public health policy; an example might be the study of the incidence of certain sorts of food-poisoning, which can have serious implications for the regulation of the sale of food products. On the face of it, because the epidemiologist ordinarily deals in previously recorded knowledge and has no clinical contact with the patient/subject concerned (indeed does not deal with individual subjects as such), the ethical dimensions of epidemiological research seem minimal or at any rate obscure.

However, even here there are some ethical problems. Clinical and medical information is still information about someone, and this has to be obtained from patient records. It is rarely practicable to obtain the permission of the patient concerned. Although the information is usually anonymised in a way that makes it ordinarily impossible to be traced back to the particular patient (and although the epidemiological researcher ordinarily has no interest in doing so), it is still proper to ask: does the information properly belong to the medical institutions or in some sense also to the patient? If the latter, then using the information without the patient's permission seems wrong. Most large epidemiological studies of existing medical records can proceed only on the assumption that the information does not belong to the patient in any meaningful sense. This assumption becomes less plausible when it concerns not only the patient's medical condition but also her social, domestic, sexual and psychological characteristics. For instance, attempts to understand people's smoking and drinking habits might benefit from exploring links with various aspects of people's domestic and employment circumstances, in which emotionally sensitive information could well play a key part. The question should always arise as to how more intimate information of this kind is obtained: was it obtained for other purposes, and if so was the subject asked whether this information – even in an anonymised and unattributable form – could later be used in research? These are pertinent questions for the REC to ask.

This problem is intensified in a second area of concern for the REC, which arises when the details of given patients are used in more than one study. If two or more studies are cross-referenced, then the combination of those two sets of information can identify an individual, particularly if she is suffering from a rare condition, even though no single set of information would in isolation be capable of identifying her.

A third area of concern arises from the implications of the knowledge obtained by the research. If the research identifies associations between a disease condition and other factors, an association moreover which is so strong as to suggest a clear causal link, then the research has an immediate bearing upon public health policy. This in itself is a good thing, of course – and exactly why the study is being carried out. However, depending on the kind of causal factors concerned (examples might include exposure to industrial toxins, for instance) it could also produce clinical obligations towards those anonymous subjects on the basis of whose medical records the knowledge was obtained. This problem may be multiplied where the disease is, as a result of the research, understood to have a genetic component; suppose for instance that a suspected genetic marker for aortic aneurysm were confirmed. In such a case, the clinical obligations now apparently extend more widely still, to the family members of subjects involved in the study. The REC will reasonably want to know what means are envisaged for contacting the research subjects (and in the case of genetically-linked conditions, their relatives) where the study reveals information that significantly affects them.

An elaboration of this problem concerns public health research using blood and tissue samples, obtained clinically for other purposes, but then subsequently anonymised and used for further screening: the most controversial recent examples concerned anonymous unlinked HIV seroprevalence screening[8]. In addition to the question of whether consent should be sought, there is the problem that the process of anonymisation made it clinically impossible to offer counselling and other support to those whose samples were identified as seropositive, since only the samples and not their human sources were identifiable.

In summary, the ethical problems of epidemiological studies are less obvious than those of clinical research, particularly because such studies typically involve no clinical contact and frequently have no clinical implications. However, when they do, does the fact that the subjects are unidentified and anonymised mean that the REC has fewer or different obligations towards them than they have towards identified and known members of the same population who are entered into clinical trials? If the obligations are different, are they less significant? The obligations must at any rate include guarantees of the preservation of anonymity (which must be especially secure when cross-referenced studies of different conditions are envisaged). Moreover, when epidemiological studies involve the analysis of unlinked (and therefore unattributable) samples of body fluids or tissues, then in consenting to such analysis the subjects must clearly understand that there is no possibility of their receiving clinical follow-up if the samples they provide test positive; the identity of the samples as 'theirs' is deliberately lost as part of the requirement of anonymising them.

3.9   Behavioural, psychological and psychiatric research

I have tried too in my time to be a philosopher; but, I don't
know how, cheerfulness was always breaking in.
(Oliver Edwards)

The field of research into psychiatric illness throws into bold relief the problems of obtaining genuine consent from participating subjects: indeed, the problems of obtaining consent are a vivid expression of the additional vulnerability of psychiatrically ill patients. Beyond this, there are characteristics of behavioural and psychological research which can be problematic even for entirely competent and healthy subjects: (i) the intention of examining people's behaviour **as such** may be challenging and threatening to the participant, since it makes aspects of the subject's personality and way of living the explicit object of examination, analysis and comment – comment which is most likely to be made in a professionalised research context from which the subject is excluded; and (ii) a minority of behavioural and psychological research concerns how people respond 'authentically' such that they are unaware of being in an experimental situation, and hence must involve at least a temporary deception of the subject. For instance, in order to observe authentic interactions among professionals (including health care professionals) or between professionals and clients, it is sometimes necessary for the researcher to conceal the fact that her subjects are being observed for fear that their behaviour would otherwise be stilted or unrepresentative[9]. Clearly it would be self-defeating for the research if the subject's permission for all aspects of it were obtained in advance – one can scarcely agree to be deceived without to some extent defeating the deception[10].

Some psychiatric research may potentially be liable to involve either or both of these problems, but in addition it is a general characteristic of psychiatric research that it can pose serious difficulties in terms of obtaining valid consents from the patients to be investigated. Psychiatric illnesses may disturb patients' understanding of what is involved, their ability to make reasoned judgements of what it is in their interests to do or to agree to, their very capacity to make decisions at all, and their ability to express or to assert or to defend their wishes, given their characteristic vulnerability in a context in which they may in some cases be receiving care and treatment **against** their expressed wishes[11].

Whilst there are many different kinds and degrees of psychiatric disturbances, many such disturbances compromise one or more of these elements of the patient's ability to exercise choice, and so getting valid consent from them is problematic; it may be difficult to interpret the responses of psychotic or profoundly depressed patients, for example. To this may be added the fact that at the present stage of knowledge psychiatric medicine is in general terms on a less secure basis, and as such is inherently more experimental, than most physical medicine[12]. Whilst this in itself might constitute a good reason why research is needed, it also raises the possibility that psychiatric research can be less securely conceived, and that the balance of risks and benefits can be less well understood, than is typically the case in clinical research in physical medicine. For instance, psychotic patients' appreciation and subsequent reporting of any unanticipated side-effects of new drugs may be coloured by the disordered nature of their thoughts; moreover there is a far less secure baseline for judging whether the new drugs themselves complicate that disorder. The predictability of the responses of psychiatric patients may also be lower. The REC will need to exercise especial scrutiny over the consent procedures and the estimations of risks and benefits in this area of research.

An obvious legal pitfall concerns the role of proxy consent[13]. It is not clear that a proxy can lawfully give consent for an adult to undergo research procedures, particularly those involving more than minimal risk. The REC needs to bear in mind here that the benefits that may be claimed for any individual arising from her participation in research are questionable – indeed this is the question (and it arises in all clinical research, not just within psychiatric research) which we shall explore below in the next section.

3.10   The 'therapeutic/non-therapeutic' distinction

This must be Fats Waller's blood. I'm getting high.
(Eddie Condon, on receiving a blood transfusion.)

It is often said that some research is inappropriate for some groups of especially vulnerable patients because it is **non-therapeutic**, that is, research from which they cannot benefit and are not intended to benefit. However, we should be careful not to assume that other research, not falling into this special category of the 'non-therapeutic', is therefore **therapeutic**, that is, beneficial or even necessarily intended to be beneficial. As Alderson has argued[14], the distinction between the therapeutic and the non-therapeutic is misleading in the context of research, because of the characteristic aims of research.

These aims, as we have already noted, concern the pursuit of new knowledge. It is not the aim of a given research project to help or cure the patients who are its subjects. Its aim is rather to find out whether the procedures and medicines being investigated will in fact help or cure patients like these; so from the point of view of the researcher at the start of the trial it is just as important to know if the patients are not in fact helped as it is to know if they **are**. Indeed, if it turns out that they are not helped, this information is just as important and from the scientific point of view just as valuable as would have been the information that they had been helped, had things turned out differently. Discovering how things turn out is what is important to the research – even though of course the reason that we wish to know this is, ultimately, in order to be able to help patients more effectively in the future. In pursuit of this discovery, neither medical science, nor the individual researcher, nor future patients will be at all helped by the spurious or accidental or misleading improvement in the condition of any of the trial subjects, if this obscures the actual effectiveness of the treatment being investigated. If, at the end of the day, we really want to be able to help more people, more reliably and more effectively, it would actually be preferable for research subjects not to get better rather than doing so for unconnected reasons which only obscured and invalidated the very results which the research is meant to produce. Furthermore, not only can we make a practical and scientific case for saying this, but at any rate the utilitarian can make a **moral** case for it as well – fewer people will be helped by unreliable research results than can be helped by reliable results. (We recall that it is for precisely this reason that, even in the case of research on the more toxic or otherwise unpleasant drugs, research trials with statistically too few subjects involved are just as unethical as trials with unnecessarily many subjects.)

Unattractive though this sounds, it is unavoidably true and it has important implications for our identifying and understanding so-called 'therapeutic' research. Research as such is not and cannot be designed to be beneficial to the research subjects involved. Its benefits – if any – concern patients in the future. If a piece of research were as such expressly designed to benefit the subjects involved, it would be very likely dishonest and unethical, since it would presuppose the very outcomes which it was meant to establish. This is not of course to deny that research subjects can get better from what is done to them in the course of research. The treatments under investigation may turn out to be highly beneficial. The point is, however, that this particular result cannot be the **aim** of honest research: honest research aims at discovering what is not yet known, without prejudice to the outcome. So if in fact some research subjects do get better, we need to be perfectly clear why this happens. If research subjects get better, they do so, not because they took part in research, but because they received a treatment which worked for them. If they are patients, they are entitled to expect to be treated in any case, and moreover to expect that the clinicians responsible for them will endeavour to make sure that they get the treatment which is believed to be best for them as individuals. This is precisely what they cannot expect in properly controlled prospective research, since the researcher is allowed no such beliefs. The research design must try to get rid of all the differences between patients which might lead to particular and non-generalisable treatment choices for them, and which might thereby prejudice or bias the results. We have already seen the elaborate statistical devices of randomisation and control groups which are employed to reduce these very dangers of bias. In agreeing to take part in any typical piece of controlled medical research, the patient agrees among other things to give up her normal expectation that she will receive the treatment believed to be best for her as an individual.

Thus if patients get better in the course of medical research, it is no thanks to the research. It is thanks to their getting medical treatment, something they were entitled to expect anyway and which, in the normal course of events outside the research context, they would expect to be more specifically tailored to their individual needs. To emphasise this point we need only recall that the usual research safeguards, which are meant to ensure that no-one in the trial is seriously jeopardised simply as a result of being in that trial, involve monitoring patients' conditions very closely: if it is suspected that they are seriously at risk by continuing in the trial they are removed from it and returned to individual clinical management: in other words, if they really need benefits which are not arising during their research participation then they are taken out of the context of research, and simply treated.

Now of course it may be objected that some people do as a matter of fact obtain benefits from being research subjects which they could not have obtained by the clinical management that they would otherwise have received: new treatments under research may, and we hope often will, offer significant improvements over the standard alternatives which are at present all that are routinely offered. In these cases, isn't it perverse to deny that the research is therapeutic with respect to those subjects who benefit from it? Once again, however, we have to acknowledge that it is not and cannot be the intention of the research as such that the subjects benefit from taking part in it: such an intention would have to rest on a firm belief in the value of the trial therapy. But if the researcher holds such a firm belief then the question of whether or not the trial patients should be offered this therapy cannot properly be a matter for research: the researcher's mind is clear on this point, and she has a simple clinical obligation to offer the therapy. The patients thus benefit, not from taking part in research but from receiving clinical treatment – as they are entitled to expect. The point may be illustrated by recalling what can happen when a particular treatment is believed to offer real benefit but is nonetheless the subject of research intended to show precisely whether or not this is true. The clamour among American AIDS sufferers to be included in the trials of AZT arose from the false belief that the experimental treatment offered help that could not otherwise be obtained – and more significantly from the fact that the novelty and rarity of the treatment meant that one could receive it only by being enrolled in the appropriate arm of a randomised controlled trial. These AIDS sufferers not only thought they could benefit from 'therapeutic' research – they thought it was the only way that they had any hope of obtaining benefit and they went to great lengths to try and secure it, including interfering with the trial's randomisation procedures, 'pooling' drugs and other subterfuges[15]. If there had been any objective grounds for these beliefs then it would have been pointless and unethical to conduct research simply in order to establish those grounds, and the AZT should have been available on criteria other than a willingness to become a research subject: research activity must not be used as a covert means of resource allocation. In the event, whatever was believed about AZT at the time, its therapeutic value proved to be illusory.

It remains true that even when we are clear that a treatment does produce benefit, we may not know how best to administer it. Thus, research may still properly be done on the matter of optimum doses, optimum timing of doses, delivery mechanisms, combinations with other therapies, and so forth – where these matters are still the subject of real uncertainty. It should be clear that those patients who benefit most from this further research do so by virtue of simply happening to receive a treatment regime that suits them, and not by virtue of any intention on the part of the researcher specifically concerning them as individual patients. In other words, here again the benefits are accidental with respect to the research itself, and cannot be claimed prospectively as a benefit of being willing to participate in the research. Such claims are all too often made in the descriptions of proposed research, and REC members need to maintain a sceptical guard against them.

There is one respect, however, in which there **is** an intentional link between participation in research and the benefits one receives – this happens when it is a matter of the design of a particular trial that the subjects do **not** benefit. Subjects simply could not receive benefit from most epidemiological or historical studies, nor, in the clinical arena, from the testing of a new drug's safety and tolerability on healthy volunteers. Research of this kind is important and necessary, and as we shall see can be properly conducted on research subjects who are competent and willing to consent to it.

3.11   Healthy volunteers and healthy controls

I came in here to help my country. I don't mind giving a reasonable amount, but a pint ...
why, that's very nearly an armful. I'm not walking around with an empty arm for anybody.

(Ray Galton and Alan Simpson, as declared by
reluctant blood donor Tony Hancock)

Healthy controls present an obvious (and in some ways straightforward) ethical challenge: by definition they do not need therapy so the research must be non-therapeutic for them **by design**. In Phase I pharmaceutical research a financial inducement is a traditionally accepted means of recruitment of healthy volunteers. With this exception it seems true that the participation of healthy controls in research on patients must rather be a matter of straightforward and genuine altruism on their part and the consent procedures must make this transparent. The REC will want to be convinced that this is so, and furthermore that the volunteers are not being asked to undergo any significant harms or risks of harms. Clearly the kinds of procedures they might be invited to undergo are heavily restricted and could not involve anything approaching surgery or significant irradiation, for instance.

Typically volunteers will be used in comparing the way the body reacts to unusual substances, irritants or allergens and they will be involved in giving samples of blood or urine. Invasive procedures such as biopsy would ordinarily be impermissible; indeed anything which is clinically contra-indicated for them is contra-indicated in the research context too, unless highly persuasive reasons can be produced, specific to the volunteers in question.

There is a complication to the question of using healthy controls where the controls in question are from one of the specially vulnerable groups identified and considered in sections 5.4, 6.6 and 6.7. A conspicuous example concerned a childhood 'glue ear' trial in which apparently innocuous skin prick tests, to be performed on healthy controls, carried a very small risk of a hyperallergic reaction necessitating the possible use of resuscitation equipment[16]. Here the risks became unjustifiable in the case of the healthy controls simply on account of the fact that as healthy children they could not benefit from the procedures themselves – in other words, the justification for putting a sick child through that risk (howsoever small) was not available in the case of children who were well. The legal position in the UK seems to be that proxy consent cannot lawfully be given for a child to take part in research which is not and cannot be therapeutic to them[17], and the position is similar in the case of incompetent adults, as we shall see in Section 6.6.

3.12   Women research subjects

I blame the women's movement for ten years in a boiler-suit.
(Jill Tweedie)

In Phases III and IV of drug development women subjects are commonly used. However, using them involves extra risks on top of those associated with the safety of the drug when administered to men; with women of childbearing age, special care has to be taken to ensure that no foetal damage may be caused in either current or prospective pregnancies. This can be done by insisting on pregnancy tests before a woman is entered into a trial and by securing her agreement to use adequate contraception during the trial and for a while after it, giving her proper warnings about the possible dangers involved in the use of experimental drugs. It might seem wiser just to bar women with childbearing potential (including nursing mothers) from such studies. Indeed, traditionally this is generally what has happened in Phase I research where women form only a very small minority of research subjects; in this phase the actions of a drug are under special scrutiny and the results of giving it to women might be distorted by interactions between it and any contraceptive drugs which they might be taking, or by variations in the way drugs are metabolised earlier and later in the menstrual cycle. So there are good scientific reasons to exclude women from studies which just test the bioavailability of a new drug or formulation: reliable results need a homogeneous group of subjects. However, there are serious objections to barring women in this way.

    We might think that it's simply wrong **in principle** to discriminate against women by denying them access to healthy volunteer trials; so long as they are given proper information and take adequate precautions, shouldn't they have equal opportunities to participate? One of the main reasons why they are relatively excluded from Phase I studies is frankly commercial: the expensive *teratology* testing (testing for damage to the foetus, which involves observing generations of animals) which is demanded of all drugs before they can be granted a product licence would, in the case of the many thousands of new drugs which have to be abandoned at the Phase I stage, be money down the drain – an understandable consideration, but hardly an answer to the principled objection.

It's also clear that many drugs are developed for use in women as well as in men. Because the drug might behave differently in the two sexes, Phase I data is needed for women as well. Since most cohorts of healthy volunteers do not include children or elderly subjects then similar considerations apply to these groups. Without specific relevant information of the sort generally provided by Phase I, giving the drug to groups who are not represented among the healthy volunteers presents real dangers. It was recently decided in the United States that half of the subjects used at Phase I should be women, so as to overcome both this problem and the general objection of principle. In the event the scientific need for homogeneity prevailed, but there was an important modification of practice. Equal subgroups of male and female subjects in Phase III are now used to see whether there are any gender differences in how a new drug is metabolised, so that appropriate dosages can be fixed; teratology testing is complete by Phase III.

Notes

1   The device rejoiced in the acronym of SQUID, standing for 'superconducting quantum interference device', a form of biomagnetometer.

2   Department of Health, Health Care Division, 'Patient satisfaction surveys', correspondence issued to Royal Liverpool Children's Hospital and others, dated 13th May 1992. A similar letter was sent at the same time to the Association of Community Health Councils for England and Wales, concerning parallel issues in Community Health Council research.

3   We are grateful to the Centre for Medicines Research for allowing us to reprint this diagram.

4   In the United Kingdom, a Clinical Trials Exemption certificate (CTX), issued by the Medicines Control Agency, is required from Phase II onwards.

5   We are very grateful to Dr John Dewhurst for providing us with the material on which this section is based.

6   Friedman, L.M., Furberg, C.D. and DeMets, D.L., *Fundamentals of Clinical Trials*, Boston: John Wright/PSG Inc. (1982, second printing), p. 66.

7   Bland, M., *An Introduction to Medical Statistics*, Oxford: Oxford Medical Publications (1988), pp. 20-21.

8   See for instance Rohen, T.E., Meade, T.W. and Mortimer, P.P., 'Monitoring the prevalence of HIV', correspondence, *British Medical Journal*, 300 (1990), p. 50; and Unlinked Anonymous HIV Surveys Steering Group, *Unlinked Anonymous HIV Prevalence Monitoring Programme, England and Wales*, London: Department of Health (1993).

9   A range of examples including some at the extreme of unacceptability are discussed in Levine, R.J., *Ethics and Regulation of Clinical Research*, 2nd edn., Baltimore/Munich: Urban & Schwarzenburg (1986), Chapter 9.

10   See the sections on 'Deception' and 'Debriefing' in: British Psychological Society, 'Ethical principles for conducting research with human participants', reprinted in *The Psychologist*, 6:1 (1993), pp. 33-5; ss. 4,5.

11   For a discussion of a number of the problems we mention here, see Fulford, K.W.M. & Howse, K., 'Ethics of research with psychiatric patients: principles, problems and the primary responsibilities of researchers', *Journal of Medical Ethics*, 19 (1993), 85-91.

12   *ibid.*, pp. 85-6

13   *ibid.*, p. 87

14   Alderson, P., 'Did children change, or the guidelines?', *Bulletin of Medical Ethics* 80 (1992), pp. 21-8; see especially pp. 23-4.

15   Institute of Medical Ethics Working Party, 'AIDS, ethics and clinical trials', *British Medical Journal*, 305 (1992), pp. 699-701.

16   For a discussion of the conflicts of interests embedded in this example, see Evans, M., 'Conflicts of interest in research on children', *Cambridge Quarterly of Health Care Ethics*, 3:4 (1994) pp. 549-559.

17   This is the advice given by the Department of Health in its *Local Research Ethics Committees*, London: Department of Health (1991); para. 4.4.

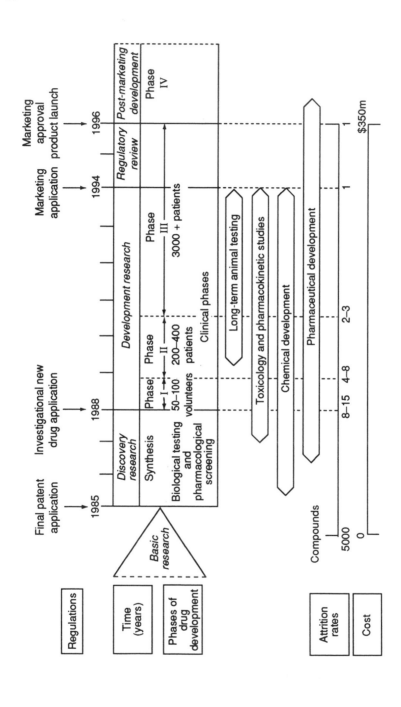

Figure 1. Discovery and development of a new medicine

(Source: Centre for Medicines Research, 1996)

Chapter Four

Experimental clinical practice

4.1   Distinguishing clinical practice from clinical research

*That is an appliance for forcing beef tea down the noses of
unsuspecting invalids. It hasn't quite found its place yet.*
(Alan Bennett)

We might think that it is a simple matter to tell apart clinical practice and
clinical research. Whilst the distinction is a necessary one, it is also subtle and
unstable. It is first of all necessary because without it we would have to choose
between on the one hand regarding all clinical practice as constituting research
and thus requiring special attention, and on the other hand regarding clinical
research as nothing more than a kind of routine clinical practice and thus
requiring no particular attention. In other words, RECs with their current brief
of examining clinical **research** would be required either to review all clinical
activity whatsoever, or to review none whatsoever – an unenviable and hopeless
choice. Faced with this choice we obviously must make the distinction between
practice and research.

However the distinction is, second, also a subtle one in the sense that the
very meaning of the word 'clinical' (deriving from ancient Greek and amounting
literally to 'at the bedside') draws our attention to the practical, often physical,
encounter with patients. Clinical research is 'clinical' just because it is a special
but nonetheless practical way of encountering patients: it is after all clinical
practice, but of a particular and special kind. The distinction works in one
direction only: all clinical research is also clinical practice, but not all clinical
practice is research; perhaps only a very small proportion is, at least in the overt
sense of 'research' with which we are concerned in this book. Generally we must

try to pick out that small proportion by examining the intentions underlying the clinical transaction: as we keep stressing, research is most clearly picked out when the **primary** intention behind it is to find out something of future importance to other patients rather than something of present importance to the patient in front of us now. Research pursues new knowledge first and foremost, rather than the good of the individual research subject.

But this brings us to the third characteristic of the distinction between clinical practice and clinical research, namely that it is unstable. By this we mean that there is a built-in uncertainty about all clinical practice, since no two patients are exactly alike: different patients have a tendency to respond differently from each other to what are on the surface comparable treatments for comparable conditions. What's more, even a given individual patient may show a variation in her response to apparently comparable interventions on different occasions, presumably owing to the presence of 'confounding' factors which are not clinically apparent other than in influencing the response in question[1]. A specialist in plastic surgery recently wrote that 'the very variable response of any individual to a standard procedure means that there is no such thing as a standard operation' and that 'every surgical act contains a research component'[2]. Of course the amount of variation need not always be significant or even noticeable. It is tied to a number of different factors including the kind of disease in question. Some disease and injury mechanisms are very well understood and can be addressed in a way that is relatively isolated from most of the personal and social characteristics of the patient (leaving aside for these purposes the question of the patient's age); this would be true of the treatment of simple bone fractures or of specific bacterial infections in a way in which it could not be true of the attempted treatment of neurological illness or psychotic illness, for instance. But once we re-admit the question of the patient's age or developmental state, very many more conditions (including bone fractures) are liable to prompt variations in individual responses. And physical diseases of a chronic nature or those with complicated multiple causal factors readily give rise to a range of individual patient responses, even when the most obvious variables have been taken into account to the best of the clinician's ability.

This means, inevitably, that even routine clinical practice involves a degree of uncertainty and a degree of experimental observation. Clinical expertise is a cumulative business, whereby each new patient encounter provides new information or data that can either confirm or confound the clinician's habits and assumptions. And since these habits and assumptions are also directed towards the future, and to the large numbers of as yet unknown, unidentified and yet-to-be-encountered patients which that future contains, then the intelligent and conscientious clinician assuredly looks to a better understanding of the good of future patients even as she reflects on the good of the patient she is treating now. In this sense, at least, all clinical practice **is** clinical research after all. And as we shall see in the next section, if this is true of clinical practice in general then it is even more true of certain areas of clinical practice where the preliminary and provisional character of clinical knowledge and technique is most obvious.

So the distinction between clinical practice and clinical research is not hard-and-fast. We could think of it as elastic, in the sense of being movable to take into account the professional and public debates over the development of emergent areas of clinical understanding (such as the techniques of *in vitro* fertilisation, for instance) so that particular groups of clinical methods and techniques gradually lose their experimental character as they become more refined and their outcomes become more predictable. Or we could think of the distinction as being 'porous', in the sense that particular instances of clinical practice can take on the character of research, as the clinician notices something about her patient, about his responses, or about the encounter between them which is striking or different or important and which, she realises, points to an adaptation in the way that she must think about (and perhaps treat) future patients like him.

Nevertheless, for all its limitations the distinction is one that must operate to underlie the role and task of RECs. Perhaps we could say that 'self-evident' research is what primarily concerns the REC – research that is conceived and undertaken and probably funded as such where it is intended, in advance of any particular clinical encounter, that from the perspective of the researcher the main purpose of the encounter is to focus on the generation of new knowledge. It is the systematic character of this intention, shown in the deliberate advance setting-up of the circumstances of the clinical encounters, that declare it to be research and to fall within the ethical responsibility of the REC. Even this way of specifying research will not convincingly exclude certain emergent areas of clinical practice such as clinical genetics, leading-edge transplantation or the newer techniques of assisted reproduction. Perhaps in recognition of this some jurisdictions have made special provision for the review and regulation of these areas of clinical practice[3], to that extent taking them out of the hands of RECs. But the prudent REC will encourage clinicians who aren't sure whether variations in their clinical practice stray into research to submit to the Committee at least a description of what they intend to do: meanwhile the prudent clinician will not wait to be asked.

4.2   New techniques in clinical practice

...nothing should ever be done for the first time.
(F.M.Cornford)

Most research protocols coming before a typical REC concern drugs[4]. There is an established recognition within the pharmaceutical industry of the case for ethical review, beyond what was until recently required by law or regulation. In the U.K. the pharmaceutical industry itself operates its own set of ethical guidelines and requirements, chiefly through the Association of the British Pharmaceutical Industry. There is no comparable arrangement on the part of the manufacturers of other kinds of medical and surgical equipment[5].

Yet a moment's thought makes it obvious that such equipment, and more importantly the clinical and surgical techniques which led to their invention and subsequent development, rest upon a process of experimentation, observation and deliberation. From the simple stethoscope to the magnetic resonance imaging scanner, from auscultation of the patient's chest to laparoscopic microsurgery, the techniques of modern clinical practice are the result of an accumulated *corpus* of observation, recording, reflection, discussion and publication over a considerable time. Sometimes this is the conscious result of a declared process[6], and sometimes it is the upshot of a virtually untraceable sequence of tacit apprenticeships and unwitting adaptations over generations of clinical practice[7]. Whatever the route, the evolution of new or revised techniques and procedures in clinical practice at the very least **implies** the conduct of clinical research upon patients – research which has historically been largely invisible to ethical review.

We say that this evolution implies clinical research for the following reasons. First, the evolution is a process of (mainly gradual) change, in which every small revision to existing practice must at some stage be carried out for the first time. Whilst this may in some instances have been entirely because there was something about a particular patient's response which indicated that the patient would be helped by doing things slightly differently, nonetheless there must always have come a point at which the variation in the practice had to be performed for the first time if it were ever to be performed at all. Second, the evolution of practice is a process in which those revisions that seemed beneficial were retained, in the hope that they might be beneficial for relevantly similar future patients. The revisions were therefore then performed for the second time (or the third, fourth or subsequent times) on patients concerning whom it was simply **supposed or conjectured** that there might be a real benefit to be had from thinking of them as being more like the patient in the original innovation than like the previous large numbers of patients treated in the old way. If the first patient to receive the modified treatment provided the occasion for forming a hypothesis, the second patient (and many subsequent patients) provided the opportunity for the hypothesis to be tested. Both the initial forming and the subsequent testing of the hypothesis look ahead to a more general future. We think that this broad account remains essentially true even when the looking forward is informal, unsystematic and when the clinician in question might more naturally have chosen the word 'hunch' than the grander-sounding 'hypothesis'.

A third reason is that whilst clinical practice is the sum of what many individual clinicians do and think, it is something which is predominantly **shared** among them. Revisions which were retained and adapted by a particular, innovative individual clinician are distributed among and adopted by her other colleagues: the new thinking becomes generalised[8]. Although clinical practice as such is a rich tapestry allowing and probably encouraging individual variation among the specific practices of individual clinicians, nevertheless its evolution implies that the convergence of different practices is more apparent, and more important, than their divergence. Even if individual clinicians freely chose to adopt all the innovations and revisions which their different practices independently brought forth, evolution relies in practice on their choosing the same revisions, and hence on their recognising those revisions, through experience, as beneficial. This could frequently be a rather informal experimental process, but it would be an experimental process for all that.

There is a fourth reason for thinking that developments in clinical practice imply a process of research, and for clinical practitioners it is probably the most convincing of all. It is that modern clinical practice claims to be founded upon science, and indeed actually to be scientific[9]. To the extent that this claim is true, the development of clinical practice must be a scientific development, a development in which each revision is stringently tested before being admitted to the body of scientific belief or understanding. In the case of knowledge about drugs and their action and effects, these revisions are accomplished within a visible research framework. Advances in many other dimensions of clinical practice are much less visibly part of a process of research; nevertheless, some kind of research process is absolutely demanded by the belief that clinical practice has its roots in science. Advances in the techniques of clinical practice must therefore largely take place either in a form of undeclared or unrecognised research (perhaps constituted by very small evolutionary changes that are generally unnoticed except with hindsight) or in a form of perfectly well recognised research that nonetheless manages to escape the attention of ethical review. The first alternative looks uncomfortable for those who profess a faith in the scientific basis of clinical practice; the second looks uncomfortable for those who believe that research on patients should be seen to be morally sound.

4.3   The problem of step-by-step innovation

The thing with high-tech is you always end up using scissors.
(David Hockney)

We have already seen how, particularly in surgery, the variation in individual responses to accepted procedures adds an experimental dimension to the 'surgical act'; we might say that research infiltrates practice whether the clinician wishes it or not. Every surgical act (perhaps every clinical act of any kind) ought in this way to contribute to what Ward has called the lower rungs of the 'ladder of research'[10]. Let's consider two examples to illustrate this important point.

Many women are troubled by urinary incontinence associated with coughing or lifting, and various surgical correctives have been tried though none has emerged as clearly the most effective. Surgeons are constantly varying their techniques and procedures, trying to simplify the surgery and make it more effective[11]. The modifications tend to happen in small steps, and many of these are never tested in a formally controlled trial at all, much less submitted for ethical review. (Because normal consents for surgery don't specify the details of the surgical techniques, surgeons often think that consent isn't needed for varying their practice in this way.) Now the abdominal wall is made up of layers including a fascial 'sheath' of thick, strong, fibrous tissue. It's possible to cut strips of this tissue to make a sling to support the neck of the bladder, helping to prevent leakage during movements such as coughing. Usually a strip about eight or so inches long is needed, and a large abdominal incision has to be made in order to get the required tissue. At first surgeons thought the sling worked by providing a continuous length of fibrous tissue, but then they found that patients who had had the operation, and who needed further surgery for unrelated reasons, did not in fact have such a continuous length of tissue. So some surgeons tried using a shorter length of fibrous tissue, anchoring it in the same places but making up the difference in length with surgical suture (stitching) – known by the somewhat laid-back nickname of 'the sling on the string'. This can be done with a much smaller surgical incision, and seems to work as well as the earlier variant.

Surgeons now think the operation really works by provoking changes in the tissues around the neck of the bladder, and that they might be able to modify the procedure still further: they might be able to take just a two-inch strip of fibrous tissue and pass it under the bladder and back without any extra lengths of suture at all. The trouble is they just don't know whether this further refinement would work as well as the current variant. Clearly the whole process of step-by-step evolution has a strong experimental element to it; but at what point in the process should the research dimension be frankly admitted, properly designed and controlled, and submitted to ethical review?

Our second example brings out this question in a life-threatening context. Neck and other spinal injuries can be either fatal or catastrophically disabling and, by reason of the very complexity and importance of the neural structures involved, the associated neurosurgery can be lengthy, complicated, exceedingly delicate and critical. The responsibility shouldered by the neurosurgeon is correspondingly heavy. Advances in equipment or techniques can make existing procedures safer, easier or more reliable, but of course they can also generate new surgical possibilities that are themselves challenging and risky. Given the potential importance of both wholly new procedures and refinements to existing practices, it seems important that each single step of innovation should be assessed properly and that its general adoption should be based on evidence.

The technique of stabilising fractures of the cervical spine (neck) using interlaminar surgical clamps (the so-called 'Halifax clamps') was first described in 1975[12]. There were long-term evaluations in the United States during the 1980s and subsequently in the U.K. The clamps in question appeared to represent a small but significant advance in the management of certain kinds of fracture, but there seems not have been the kind of inital, systematic and controlled testing that would be routine in the introduction of a new drug[13]. After an initial period some practitioners noticed post-operative failures in the clamps, recorded their own experiences and then launched a nationwide survey. This survey showed that the clamp had a failure rate of about 20% when used at the critical fracture sites (the high cervical vertebrae), the very sites where failure of stabilisation could be fatal[14,15]. Following the publication of this survey the clamps were temporarily withdrawn and were put back onto the market only after extensive alterations had been made to the design[16].

Whatever assessment process led to the initial marketing of these clamps seems incomplete in both practical and ethical terms. The design modifications which were necessary to make the clamps safe in use were identified and put in place only **after** the clamps had been introduced into neurosurgical practice. Before those modifications, but nevertheless whilst on the market and in surgical use, the clamps' failures made them significantly unreliable and potentially lethal. In effect, the research process leading to an effective, safe and usable fastening was not complete when the clamps were first marketed, but was subsequently conducted on the general population of neck-fracture patients in ordinary neurosurgical practice. This part of the research — clearly necessary, as it turned out, for the production of a safe and reliable design – was effectively invisible and unacknowledged. Indeed we must assume that it was unintended by the manufacturers, who presumably believed, or at any rate hoped, that the design as originally marketed was adequate. (We must assume this because the only alternative is to suppose that the manufacturers intended that the testing of the clamps should be largely performed in this unacknowledged way, and it would be a very serious matter indeed to suggest that something so clearly and so gravely wrong was done on purpose.) But of course if we do assume that this part of the research process was unintended by the manufacturers, it is almost certain that neither the surgeons who used the clamps nor the patients on whom the clamps were used knew or believed that they were engaged in clinical research either. This is precisely what makes this part of the research invisible and unacknowledged, and it is these two features which illustrate the dangers of step-by-step innovation; no single step may be sufficiently obvious to be recognised as an instance of research, and hence research is carried out by default – on patients who do not realise that they are research subjects, by practitioners who do not realise that they are clinical investigators, and the whole thing without the benefit of an ethical review process to consider evidence about the relative risks and benefits of the innovation or to ensure appropriate consent procedures.

Someone might of course object to this conclusion. They might deny that the dividing line between clinical practice and clinical research has been improperly crossed. They could begin by pointing out that step-by-step innovation is first of all necessary since in many innovative processes no single step is possible without all of its predecessors. They could go on to claim that front-line practitioners are the only people who can properly judge the risks and benefits of each new step, and only in the context of trying it out in their general clinical practice; and that (as we have already agreed) there is an inevitably experimental aspect of virtually all clinical practice, an aspect which is more obviously visible in some clinical areas than in others precisely because of the provisional state of knowledge and expertise in those areas. Finally our objector might conclude that step-by-step innovation can be accompanied by a perfectly satisfactory consent process, provided that clinicians are open with their patients about the incomplete nature of their knowledge and about their intention to try out the latest techniques and equipment.

What this objection does is both to challenge the hard-and-fast division between research and practice, and to claim that even if such a division can be shown to have been crossed, it can be morally acceptable to cross it given the protections of the usual consent processes. There is something to be said for both parts of this view. Our concern throughout this chapter springs from our recognising how blurred the distinction between research and practice can be; and our complaint about the invisible or unacknowledged nature of some research is of course answered in full, if a consent process makes the research both visible and recognised by the parties to it[17]. But there is an important difference between, on the one hand, obtaining the consent of a patient to undergo an innovative or unproven procedure which is nonetheless – so far as can be known – likely to represent the best available treatment for him, and on the other hand obtaining the consent of a patient to undergo an unproven procedure as a part of the very process of discovering its safety and efficacy. This second consent is a consent to take part in research, and must be presented as such. Ethical review procedures are there to make sure that this happens, and indeed that the existing evidence concerning the safety and efficacy of the new technique is sufficiently compelling and sufficiently favourable to justify inviting patients to undergo it at all. And acknowledged research on patients must be submitted to the scrutiny of an REC. But this happened only retrospectively in the case of certain applications of the Halifax clamp. As things turned out, at the time when it really mattered – that is,

prospectively – no-one seems to have recognised that the relevant research process was incomplete and still under way.

4.4   Research by stealth?

When I was in Venice I thought that perhaps masked naked men, orgies and
unlimited spying are an accompaniment of maritime powers in decline.
(Nancy Mitford)

We've seen that the distinction between clinical practice and clinical research is sometimes unclear.   Sometimes this unclarity is exploited to enable questionable procedures to avoid the ethical review process.   Of course people may disagree over when this actually happens, but then the decision about whether ethical review is necessary ought to taken by someone other than the researcher.

Consider for instance the observation of suspected child-abusing parents by covert video surveillance[18].   It is a case over which people have got into precisely that sort of disagreement;   whichever view one might eventually take of the practice in question, it illustrates well the problems we are considering.   Now of course good clinical practice requires a critical evaluation of procedures and outcomes.   In this sense the boundaries of knowledge are pushed back through step-by-step learning in practice.   However, the quest for new knowledge might involve departures from established practice that are so considerable that research goals replace, or at least compete with, ordinary diagnostic or therapeutic goals.   Where this happens then the subjects of that practice have rights and needs which should be respected and protected by an independent assessment of its invasiveness, of any breaches of privacy or threats to their well-being and so on.

In the case in point the practitioners wanted to find out whether there was a correlation between multi-channel recordings of various physiological functions in children suffering apnoeic attacks that were due to natural causes and the recordings of children who suffered similar attacks that were due to deliberately imposed upper airway obstruction.   They wanted to test the hypothesis that, given certain instrumentation they had developed, they would be able to tell from reading the recorded traces alone when a violent attack upon a child was occurring.   To find out, they had to compare traces recorded in cases where there were undisputedly natural causes on the one hand and violent attacks on the other.   Of course the need to detect life-threatening child abuse on the part of certain parents also gave an opportunity to obtain criminal evidence of deliberate child abuse, so long as the parents in question remained ignorant of the observers.   The practitioners arranged for the child to stay in hospital, accompanied by the suspected parent, in a specially prepared room which was subjected to round-the-clock video surveillance.   The surveillance continued for many days in the hope of obtaining incontrovertible evidence of an attack upon the child which would stand up in a court of law. Once begun, an attack had to be allowed to go on long enough for a suitable video record to be made and for suitable traces to be recorded to test the hypothesis. This inevitably meant deliberately exposing the child to possible harms – and exposing the abusing parent to unusual and novel pressures to commit the attack. Presented as a research project in this way we suspect that most ethical review committees would have considerable difficulty in approving the procedure.

The practitioners in question, however, described the procedure in a different way. They were engaged in 'vital clinical work' protecting the health of the child in avoiding future life-threatening attacks on the child by demonstrating the cause of its apnoea and removing that cause, with the help of the courts who would separate the child from the offending parent.

It is not our purpose here to rehearse arguments for and against one or other description of the procedures in question, though this has been done in some detail elsewhere[19]. Rather, the example illustrates how what some may regard as an intrusive and dangerous research procedure, which neglected the rights and welfare of research subjects, might be presented instead as clinical practice calling for no independent opinion about its propriety. It seems to us that where such a disagreement reasonably occurs then the matter ought to be discussed with the chairperson of an appropriately constituted REC to determine, independently of the research enthusiasm of the practitioner, whether the practice is in fact so exceptional and contains such a significant research element as to require full discussion by an independent review committee.

Notes

1   Observing and grappling with these variations inevitably played an important part in the development of modern understandings of disease. For an engaging discussion of this see Dubos, R., *Mirage of Health*, New Brunswick: Rutgers University Press (1959), Chapter 4.

2   Ward, C., 'Research into surgery', in Consumers for Ethics in Research (CERES), *CERES News*, 18 (1995), pp. 2-7; see particularly p. 2.

3   In the U.K., they are the subject respectively of the recommendations of the Clothier Report, the Unrelated Live Transplants Regulatory Authority and the Human Fertilisation and Embryology Authority.

4   This is our experience from personal participation in two N.H.S. RECs and one independent REC, and is confirmed by the reported experience of members of many other RECs.

5   The national training conferences for chairmen and members of British RECs, which we have co-organised and co-facilitated for a number of years, attracts participants from the pharmaceutical industry but not from manufacturers of medical or surgical equipment.

6   Inevitably this is most readily seen in the modern high-tech medicine. In Chapter Thirteen we will discuss the idea of 'impact assessment' of new technology: there we consider the excellent study of a specific example, the computed tomography (CT) scanner, which is to be found in Stocking, B. and Morrison, S.L., *The Image and the Reality: a Case Study of the Impacts of Medical Technology*, London: Nuffield Press (1978).

7   Midwifery practice, increasingly vocal in its resistance to being subsumed under the medical category, is an example of a 'craft' that has evolved according to this way. And the evolution need not always be progressive; Ward says that 'surgeons may make claims about clinical judgement when they are simply guessing or obediently repeating their predecessors' mistakes'. Ward, *op. cit.*, p.3.

8   This is as true in terms of theoretical understanding as it is in terms of clinical technique. The emergence and general acceptance of the germ theory of disease, subsequently driving both clinical practice and research, is a case in point.

9   See for instance the view of Rudolf Virchow, quoted in Bynum, W.F., *Science and the Practice of Medicine in the Nineteenth Century*, Cambridge: Cambridge University Press (1994), p. 118.

10   Ward, *loc. cit.*

11   We are grateful to Mr Simon Emery, Consultant Obstetrician and Gynaecologist at Singleton Hospital, Swansea, for giving us a detailed description of this example.

12   Tucker, H.H., 'Method of fixation of subluxed or dislocated cervical spine below C1-C2', *Canadian Journal of Neurological Sciences*, 2 (1975), 381-2.

13   While the clamp's use in the lower spine proved to be safe and reliable, by 1992 – 17 years after its introduction – there had still been only 46 **reported** cases of its use in the high cervical vertebrae. See Statham, P., O'Sullivan, M. and Russell, T., 'The Halifax interlaminar clamp for posterior cervical fusion – initial experience in the United Kingdom', *Journal of Neurosurgery*, 32(3) (1993), pp. 396-9.

14   *ibid.*

15   Russell T, personal communication, 8th January 1995.

16   *ibid.*

17   There is of course more to be said about whether arguments based solely on considerations of consent can settle anything by themselves. See Chapter Six, especially section 6.7.

18   For a fuller discussion of this case see Evans, D., 'Investigating life-threatening child abuse and Munchausen's syndrome by proxy', *Journal of Medical Ethics*, 21:1 (1995), pp. 9-13.

19   *ibid.*

Chapter Five

Balancing risks and benefits

5.1 Problems of identification

All right, have it your way – you heard a seal bark.
(James Thurber)

What count as the risks and the benefits of a particular piece of research? We generally assume that the risks concern what happens to the research subjects during and (reasonably) soon after the trial period, whereas the benefits concern future, as yet hypothetical, patients. Whilst this is basically true, it is by no means easy to specify the risks and benefits at all precisely. To begin with, there is the problem that 'risk' can be understood in either of two different ways: as a degree of likelihood (or probability) that something will happen, or as the kind and severity of harm which lies behind certain kinds of situation. When people ordinarily speak of the risks of clinical research, presumably some combination of the two is intended: that is, a given likelihood of incurring a given kind and severity of harm. When the REC studies the risks of a proposed piece of clinical research, these two components need to be distinguished.

The assumption, that the risks are exclusively those which are undergone by the research subject, rules out consideration of the socio-economic risks arising from the adoption of new resource patterns which are occasionally encouraged by therapeutic innovations (e.g. infertility treatments, diagnostic scanning, the identification of new diseases, or the emergence of effective but highly expensive drugs or surgical techniques). This may not formally be the REC's business, but in a situation of scarcity groups of patients who are not under consideration may in the future have their access to health care restricted as a result of moving resources towards patients who are presently the focus of research interest. (It is worth recording that at least one U.K. Health Authority, West Glamorgan HA in South

Wales, has recognised these implications and established a 'Purchaser Advice' ethics committee to consider the ethical implications of its policy and planning decisions[1]. Whilst these do not exclusively concern the impact of research and development, they do obviously include it.) Another qualification of the assumption that only research subjects face the risks of clinical research arises when it is seen that the assumption rules out concern for the health, safety and financial indemnity of the researchers themselves, something that plainly **is** the REC's business. Lastly, the character of the intended benefits even for individual future patients can sometimes be questioned, as in the case of research which is meant to further the development of genetic screening kits for home use: a topical example, an over-the-counter genetic test for **susceptibility** to breast cancer, seems to offer benefits that are more Faustian than clinical. RECs are meant to consider the importance of the questions which specific research addresses, but they have no clear mandate to obstruct developments which they might find socially questionable.

Even granting the assumption that the risks of research bear basically upon the research subjects themselves, we must somehow distinguish those risks which essentially arise from the fact that the procedures constitute research, from the risks which arise from the standard treatment alternative which the subject would otherwise expect. Having picked out general predicted risks of this kind, then further problems arise from the difficulties of predicting individual variations in response. We obviously need to be able to tell whether the occurrence of adverse reactions is a risk accruing to the research *per se* or to the unforeseeable combination of the research and a particular atypical and unpredictable subject. The authors were once involved in reviewing a Phase I trial in which an apparently adverse event occurred in the form of an arrhythmia in one of the subjects. Once the tell-tale trace was picked up the subject was immediately withdrawn from the trial and observed by a physician to ensure that his ECG traces remained normal. Immediate steps were taken to find out whether the arrhythmia was related to the trial drug. The other subjects were kept under close surveillance, while the subject in question was monitored by means of a twenty-four hour Holter ECG device. The trace from that monitor showed that the subject had a naturally occurring second degree Type One heart block, and so the arrhythmia was considered to be 'normal' (i.e. to be expected) for the individual in question. Because it showed itself only occasionally the condition had not been detected in the medical checks run prior to the trial. These problems are exactly parallel to the problems of crediting research procedures with the benefits of the treatment involved – it seems only fair to absolve research as such from responsibility for any risks which the patient would face in any case, such as from his ordinary course of treatment. When brand new treatments are being tested (and particularly when their toxicity is one of the explicit objects of study) and when moreover it is only in the course of the research that a patient would be exposed to such a treatment, then it seems fair to attribute the risks of the treatment to the research process.   But most research is not like this. So when, as is more usual, different variations of existing treatments are being compared, then we need to identify what risks arise actually from the process of research itself: essentially, these risks arise from the problems of allocating (and perhaps randomising) patients to receive less than optimal (or even no) treatment. That is, in the more usual cases, the risks of research are more to do with the possibility of patients missing out on benefits which they need, than they are to do with undergoing especially risky therapies which they do **not** need. Research of this last kind would be ethically suspect by that very token. Attributing risks to the research process as such is a tricky business (and must be done with as much care and scruple as we should employ when attributing benefits).

On the benefit side, the hypothetical nature of future benefits brings obvious problems of identification. One concerns the supposition that we will be able to tell what proportion of any clinical improvement in appropriate future patients can be attributed to the results of the present research;   another is the question of whether initially unforeseen or secondary beneficial effects of the treatment under investigation should ultimately be included in the balance. Again there are a number of supposed benefits which arguably ought not to be allowed to count, including the ordinarily expected therapeutic gain for the research subjects from standard treatment, or any developments in research expertise and facilities, or the advancement of reputations and research profiles, or the various intangibles such as the 'amount' of altruism in society, and so forth.

Even more difficult is the question of whether certain phenomena can generally even be understood as benefits or risks, in view of the fact that they may be very differently assessed by given individuals (a problem especially acute in psychiatric research where depression, for instance, can lead to paradoxical evaluations of risks as benefits, and *vice versa*; we discuss such a case in section 5.4).

5.2   Unequal shares: the distribution of risk and benefit

I long ago came to the conclusion that all life is 6 to 5 against.
(Damon Runyon)

Morally speaking, one of the most striking characteristics of clinical research is obviously that those who undergo its attendant risks are usually not those who will obtain its benefits, 'therapeutic' research notwithstanding. We can bring this out by considering the different probabilities of risks and benefits. The risks are generally predictable, first in the sense that it can be anticipated what sort of harms may occur (for instance, specific side effects of drugs such as the stomach irritation arising from certain kinds of anti-inflammatory drugs, or the potential embarrassment or disturbance arising from certain kinds of questionnaires, or the physical discomfort or distress arising from various investigative procedures such as biopsies) and also, second, in the sense that some idea of the likelihood or probability can be given for the occurrence of many of these harms (ranging from very low chances of, for instance, hyperallergic reactions in the case of allergy tests, to the virtual certainty of, for instance, discomfort or even moderate distress arising in the performance of gastro-endosocopy). We know, furthermore, who it is that is at risk – we can know by face and by name, if necessary, the people who confront these harms, because they are the reseach subjects who have been recruited.

By contrast, the people who will get the benefit of the research are hypothetical: they are almost invariably unknown to us and furthermore we cannot know with any certainty that anyone ever will benefit. (If the benefits were certain, there would be no point in undertaking research in order to establish them, and it would of course be quite unethical to do so.) Of course we hope that people will benefit, and in large numbers. However, given the time involved in the development of new drugs in particular, it is clear that these hypothetical beneficiaries are not likely to be at all the same people as those who bear the risks of the research.

Two things arise from this unequal distribution: first, those who volunteer to be research subjects are to be admired for their generosity; second, they deserve all the protection that we can give them, and once we have recognised this, then at least one compelling rationale for the ethical review process is already given without more needing to be said. Plainly, one source of protection is to restrict the risks involved in proposed clinical research, and we regard it as a key rôle of the REC to ensure to its satisfaction that the risks are indeed minimal. This idea in itself needs some examination.

5.3   The idea of 'minimal risk'

> *Opera is when a guy gets stabbed in the*
> *back and instead of bleeding, he sings.*
> (Ed Gardner)

The point of appealing to the idea of 'minimal risk' lies in assuming that risks which are minimal can be morally acceptable in a way in which any greater degree of risk could not. Admittedly there is more to the acceptability of a risk than this, since greater risks might be justified in some circumstances – for instance, where the research subjects were very sick, and needed at least the chance of benefitting from novel treatments which were known or suspected to have serious side effects. Nevertheless it is attractive to hope for some idea or interpretation of 'minimal risk' which will allow us to distinguish between research which is ethically acceptable and research which is not. Assuming that such an interpretation could be found, then we shall take the idea of 'minimal risk' to be a moral benchmark for clinical research. Whilst there are many contexts in which autonomous adults can choose to undertake more-than-minimal risks (sport is an obvious example), clinical research ought perhaps not to be among them. The main reason for thinking this is that we should distinguish between the degree of risk someone might privately undergo in an activity of his choice, and the degree of risk it is appropriate for a professional or other public figure to **invite** a patient to contemplate. We shall say more about vulnerable groups in the next section, and more about the obstacles to and the limitations on valid consent in Chapter 6.

If we accept that the idea of minimal risk ought indeed to be our benchmark, then two specific interpretations of the idea of 'minimal risk' have been suggested as a template for identifying and evaluating the risks involved in a research proposal. (These ideas have been well explored by Nicholson[2].) The two interpretations are to some extent tied to the distinction between so-called 'therapeutic' and 'non-therapeutic' research, discussed previously:

5.3.1   When research is avowedly non-therapeutic, we could say that the risks are minimal if the research procedures involve no foreseeable harms which are either more likely, or more severe, than those which one could meet in everyday life. It is accepted that daily living involves a certain amount of risk, after all. However, a problem with this interpretation of 'minimal risk' is that different people's daily lives vary enormously; are the relevant clinical risks to be compared with the typical daily life of a schoolteacher, or of a long-distance lorry-driver, or of a steelworker, or of a librarian? (If a schoolteacher, then in an urban secondary school or in a rural primary school? And so on.)

The variety of individual risks could be multiplied indefinitely (for instance even leisure activities range from hang-gliding to reading romantic fiction), and it will be hard to produce a convincing account of a standard 'package' of everyday risk. (This is deliciously illustrated by one of the more memorable gags from the black comedy devoted to the eponymous rock group Spinal Tap, in which it is reported that one of a series of luckless drummers attached to the group has been killed 'in a bizarre gardening accident'.) Neither will it be easier to apply such a template to the great variety of risks to be found in the clinical setting, which range from the possible physical harms of medical investigations to the possible emotional or psychological harms of contemplating, for instance, genetic risk factors or perhaps latent sexuality.

5.3.2   The main alternative conception of 'minimal risk' is more promising, particularly as it directly faces up to the problem of which benefits and which risks should be laid at the door of the research procedures themselves. In the case of research labelled as therapeutic, 'minimal risk' might reasonably be held to be risk which is no greater (that is, which refers to harms which are no more severe and no more likely) than the risks to be undergone anyway in the treatment which the research subject would receive were she not in the research project. If the research involves no additional risk beyond these, then it meets the requirements of 'minimal risk' and furthermore does so in a way which clarifies which outcomes (be they beneficial or harmful) properly arise from carrying out the research itself. If it does involve additional risks then at any rate those risks can be said to be non-minimal (as for instance where the trial design requires randomisation to placebo groups, or additional investigative procedures) and the REC will have at least a conception of the degree of risk which comes from the research itself – and, furthermore, some way of gauging whether it represents a morally significant increase in the risks already facing the patient. This is the sort of thing that RECs should routinely discover when they examine proposed research, and a specific enquiry on this matter could usefully be made a part of the REC's *pro-forma* application requirements – something we shall explore in Chapter Nine. An important related point is that this interpretation of 'minimal risk' enables research subjects to be invited to take part in the research on the basis of a clear understanding of the sort of risk that participation will pose to them. As such, this second conception of 'minimal risk' is one which can equally well be applied to straightforward non-therapeutic research as well. Patients in openly non-therapeutic research can expect no benefit to arise from the trial itself. However, the REC can – indeed must – judge whether the additional risks of the research, when compared to the existing risks of treatment which the patient is undergoing, are nonetheless sufficiently small that a patient could reasonably be invited to contemplate them.

In the case of healthy volunteers or controls, who of course simply would not be receiving any medical treatment of the kind proposed were they not in taking part in the research, it is easy enough just to identify what the risks of taking part in the research actually are. Quite simply, **all** the risks involved are due to taking part in the research. Furthermore these risks can be spelled out clearly. Picking out the risks is not, of course, in itself to discover whether they are minimal. But it's not clear that either of the two interpretations of 'minimal risk' would help us. Whether or not the risks compared favourably with the risks of a supposedly typical daily life is likely to remain as obscure as ever; however, the REC will at least have the material it needs to attempt a judgement as to whether the risks are unacceptably high.

5.4   Special cases and special groups

Poets are almost always bald when they get to be about forty.
(John Masefield)

There are some groups of research subjects who are in need of special protection (as we shall see in more detail below in our discussion of proxy consent in sections 6.6 and 6.7 below). The frail elderly, the mentally impaired, younger or less mature children, the physically vulnerable such as those with severe handicap, chronic pain or terminal illness, those with lowered consciousness, those with clinical depression and so on may require assistance in identifying and assessing the risks and benefits to them of a particular procedure; some of these groups may need help simply in understanding them. Furthermore, being in one of these groups may complicate or even obscure the question of what the risks and benefits actually are.

Medical research on children, for instance, involves the possibility of developmental harms: the long-range consequences of an adverse event might be far more serious for a child than for an adult, not simply in terms of the length of time that they have to be endured, but also in terms of their gravity. For instance, the toxic metabolites of certain drugs might accumulate in tissues which are growing and developing, and could thus cause much greater damage – interfering with proper growth, for example – than would be the case with an adult. (A related phenomenon accounts for the greater susceptibility of children to intellectual impairment from environmental exposure to lead poisoning, and provided one of the strongest arguments in favour of reducing lead pollution from vehicle exhaust fumes.) It's true of course that the hoped-for benefits of therapeutic advances might, in children, be potentiated in exactly the same way. All we can say is that here again, the benefits of research are characteristically more hypothetical than are the harms. Again the child is at risk of particular psychological harms from the uneasy mixture of intentions that characterise clinical research. This leads us naturally to consider the special place that trust has in the life of a child: a child has no alternative but to trust those responsible for her care – whether or not they are able to meet that responsibility. She will naturally believe that her carers will always do what is best for her: if she is healthy, she would not expect to be asked to take unnecessary medicines, whilst if she is sick she would not expect to be asked to undergo anything but the treatment which is best for her needs. The specially intense problems of using healthy children as controls, or sick children in the placebo arm of a controlled trial, arise from the central rôle that trust has in a child's life. Any apparent violation of that trust risks causing unpredicatable psychological harms.

Trust may play an equally central rôle in the lives of other dependent groups of research subjects: the declining elderly, the mentally ill or the mentally impaired for instance. It is precisely because these groups rely (to varying degrees) on other people, to represent their interests and to take decisions on their behalf, that they too are vulnerable to the risk of psychological harms associated with their dependency. Beyond this, each group faces additional, characteristic risks. If it is true, as we earlier suggested, that psychiatric and psychological medicine has an essentially less secure and more experimental standing than many branches of physical medicine, then expressly experimental work in this context is likely to be correspondingly less predictable in its effects. Additionally, we noted that psychiatric and psychological research implicitly investigates not merely how people are but also **what** they are, and as such is unusually threatening.

These groups' vulnerability arises in part from difficulties concerning their ability to make their own choices, but other patient groups' vulnerabilities can arise simply from their physical condition. For instance, those who are chronically ill or disabled may encounter harms from ordinary procedures which would be unnoticed by other patients; anyone with chronic joint pain might find even passive flexion of limbs to be painful. And their physical dependency on others can mean that simply undergoing **additional** procedures for research purposes extends and reinforces their reliance on other people for help with things that the rest of us would regard as nothing more than a minor inconvenience: we need think only of the provision of urine or faecal samples, for instance, in this connection. Sufferers of very rare conditions, or conditions which are still in the process of attracting general medical recognition (myalgic encephalomyelitis would be an example) may be especially targeted for research purposes again and again. The very fact of being constantly identified by their debilitating condition may in itself amount to a further psychological ordeal, as well as devalue them as people. The elderly as a group, and particularly the frail elderly, can face many extra vulnerabilities. It has been reported that elderly patients are characteristically deferential to clinical requests including requests to take part in research; discussing their concerns with survey research on elderly patients, Strain and Chappell record that 'since these participants generally "do as directed" by staff, the task of obtaining consent [for the research] was relatively easy'[3]. They may have an acute sense of personal dignity and propriety that can easily and unwittingly be violated in ways quite unanticipated by the rest of us – a problem that arises just as easily in standard clinical practice, of course. Moreover the frail elderly may be able to benefit from research in only a relatively limited number of ways, depending on their underlying condition. Indeed, taking this concern nearer to its conclusion, the meaning and scope of 'benefit' for the terminally ill is obviously questionable. They may still be willing – and might even want – to take part in research for the benefit of future patients, but we should be very clear about when, if at all, research on such groups offers them anything more beneficial than simply undergoing additional medical procedures and attention.

Lastly we come to the problem of distinguishing harms from benefits. The clinically depressed, for instance, may form odd or even paradoxical interpretations of harm and benefit, such as in seeing the risks of certain adverse events in a favourable rather than an unfavourable light. A striking example is reported from clinical practice rather than research, but it makes the point. A middle-aged woman, suicidal from her serious depressive illness, was asked to consent to undergo electro-convulsive therapy (ECT). She was told about the benefits that it was hoped the therapy might produce, and she was told also about the risks of possible side effects and of serious adverse events. Among these was the statistical possibility of death. She asked what the probability was of this happening, and was told that there was one chance in three thousand. 'I hope I'm the one' was her response[4].

This case is a vivid one; however we can readily appreciate it. Psychiatric illnesses are frequently characterised by the sufferer's expressing judgements which other people regard as disordered. Sometimes the disorder appears to lie in failures of reasoning, but in other cases it is exhibited in what other people regard as bizarre or paradoxical values and beliefs. The assessment of risks and benefits reflects personal values in all cases, but the assessment is specially complicated in the case of particularly vulnerable groups whose sense of their own scale of values may be unusual, incompletely formed, imperfectly understood by others, or beyond their own ability to express.

5.5   Ideas, incommensurables and the question of quantification

The chief end of Man is to frame general ideas... and no general idea is worth a damn.
(Oliver Wendell Holmes Jr)

Weighing risks and benefits is, according to the official *IRB Guidebook*,

> ....the major ethical judgement that [RECs] must make in reviewing research proposals. The risk/benefit assessment is not a technical one valid under all circumstances;   rather it is a judgement that often depends upon prevailing community standards and subjective determinations of risk and benefit. Consequently different [RECs] may arrive at different assessments of a particular risk/benefit ratio.[5]

This is a considerable understatement. The problem is not simply that, given some agreed numerical balance between twelve units of risk and thirteen units of benefit, different Committees are entitled to disagree over whether the one extra unit of benefit is decisive (though this would certainly be true). Much more intractable is the problem that risks and benefits cannot be parcelled up in this way – we all know that we have never heard of such units of risk and benefit, and a little reflection will tell us that we are never likely to either, at least in any remotely persuasive terms. Even when the probability of a given harms or a given benefits actually occuring can be identified (itself inevitably a statistical generalisation that can be no more than approximate and that may or may not be true in a given instance) we are left with the problem of putting a number on the size or significance of the harm or the benefit. But this is almost entirely a matter of personal evaluation, unlikely ever to be amenable to more than a loose, rough-and-ready agreement about whether one type of harm is broadly speaking more serious than another type.

Confining ourselves for the moment simply to the comparison of different harms, and taking an example that would be unusually clear-cut in the context of clinical reseach, it is highly unlikely that we could get people to agree about whether partial impairment of sight were worse than partial impairment of hearing or of mobility, since the significance of these things depends on which highly-valued activities in different people's lives require the full use of these different faculties. Whether such impairments were temporary or permanent might markedly alter the importance attached to them by different individuals. Moreover, it would be still more difficult to get people to agree on the relative seriousness of the more typical harms arising in clinical research, such as (in the case of drug side effects) periods of nausea, dizziness, lassitude, sweating, trembling or headaches, or (in the case of surgical interventions) peri- and post-operative complications ranging from localised pain and stiffness to specific paralyses, let alone more permanent loss of specific function. Put crudely, it depends on what different people differently fear. And even where agreement could be obtained (as it might, but certainly need not be, over whether for instance recurrent diarrhoea were preferable to permanent stiffness or loss of dexterity in one's hands), that agreement would concern only the relative importance of a restricted number of different general harms and not their absolute weight on any comprehensive numerical scale.   However, in many or perhaps most cases, the attempt at comparison will strike us as fairly meaningless.

If this is true within the category of risk or within the category of benefit, it is even more starkly true when trying to compare, across these categories, the significance of a possible harm with the significance of a possible benefit: how much pain, confusion or nausea is worth how much reduced inflammation and increased mobility? Worse still, and entirely characteristic of the future-orientated outlook of clinical research, how much of that harm as incurred today by volunteer Jones is worth how much of that benefit as (hopefully) enjoyed in four years' time by patient Smith?

It's hard to resist the conclusion that comparisons such as these are to all intents and purposes meaningless – yet they are at the core of any supposedly 'objective', systematic attempt to quantify and to weigh risks and benefits. They seem simultaneously to be a moral necessity and an intellectual outrage. (Not all commentators agree, however, and a heroic attempt to produce a convincing risk/benefit equation for a piece of clinical research has been undertaken by Nicholson[6]. We think the attempt fails, however, because at the root of its undoubtedly impressive calculations it relies on an artificial scale of illness valuation whose derivation seems to us to be questionable both in practical and in theoretical terms[7].) It is ultimately because these things cannot be converted into numbers at all, rather than because of some merely accidental failure of different people to add the 'numbers' up correctly, that the REC's judgement will be a subjective one. But if this is a difficulty for ethical review, we might as well recognise now that it is one which no amount of ingenuity will ever enable us to avoid.

5.6   Subjective judgements, social norms: 'Would you let your daughter ... ?'

Actresses will happen in the best regulated families.
(Oliver Herford)

We might be tempted to suppose that, because there is no 'correct' answer to the problem of weighing the risks and benefits of a piece of proposed research, and because all judgements about the actual balance are subjective, no-one's judgement is any better than anyone else's and we should simply leave the decision up to the individual preference of the research subject. In particular, we might think the REC can have no expertise and hence no authority to approve or disapprove research on the grounds of the balance between risks and benefits, since if all judgements are equally subjective then there is no such thing as expertise in this area.

But this conclusion should be resisted, for several reasons. First of all there is the assessment of whether the possible harms of a particular piece of research are more than minimal, as defined by comparison with the possible harms of the relevant standard clinical treatment. For any given harm, the probabilities can be roughly compared; furthermore for a given procedure, any new or additional harms can be identified. The REC, provided it has appropriate experience, and access to suitable advice, is particularly well placed to make this assessment. It is better placed than patients since it can draw on knowledge of what a wide range of clinical treatments actually involve, and it is better placed than the clinicians and researchers themselves because its distance and independence from the situations concerned enables it to make the comparison among treatments dispassionately, and without any liability (however unwitting) to ignore or under-regard relevant details.

Second, the REC can come to a collective, rather than simply individual (and hence possibly idiosyncratic), judgement about whether any additional possible harms ought to be classed as substantial – for instance, whether they are likely to be regarded as substantial by very many patients. The fact that some patients might, individually, not happen to disvalue a particular harm has no bearing on whether patients in general ought to be **invited** to hazard encountering that harm in the course of taking part in the research. We shall explore this point further in section 6.8.

Third, and connected with this, the REC should, over the period of its functioning, accumulate the clinical and other experiences of its members as to which clinical harms are in fact seriously regarded and where possible avoided by many or most patients. The fact that these harms cannot be put into even an ordinal scale, let alone a cardinal one (still less into the same ordinal or cardinal scale as some other people's benefits) does not mean that they cannot be identified as significant harms to which patients should or should not be exposed, even in the course of important medical research. By so doing, the REC exercises its representative function of reflecting preferences which have been and continue to be expressed by the patient population for whom it has responsibility. In this sense the official *IRB Guidebook*'s reference to 'prevailing community standards' does have a point to it. This is the kind of idea which, while tied to particular times, places and attitudes, is nonetheless valid in those contexts. It is also the reason why – as we shall see later in Chapter Twelve – even when the general ethical appropriateness of multi-location research may be considered elsewhere than by the REC, it is the local Committee which should have the final decision as to whether it is locally appropriate to recruit members of its own clinical population into that research.

Fourth, the REC is not charged with establishing whether the benefits that are anticipated from a particular piece of research are optimal or even particularly substantial; indeed it is not clear from the U.K. Department of Health's *Guidelines* how benefits are to be assessed at all, beyond the REC's being in some sense satisfied that the risks to the research subject are justified either by the expected benefit to himself or by the expected 'collective benefit'[8]. Since this judgement is precisely what we are trying to elucidate, the Department's advice is not very helpful. It does seem, however, that there is no notion of optimal or maximal benefit that can correspond with the notion of minimal risk. Accordingly, the REC is entitled to be satisfied first and foremost whether the risk is indeed minimal, and in the final section of this chapter we shall consider some practical steps which can help ensure that it is. We think that it is only where the risk is **not** minimal, in the sense defined above by reference to the risks of standard treatment, that the weight of benefit carries the chief burden of justifying the research. Thus in a large proportion of the research which an REC will consider, the risk/benefit assessment need not stray into those conceptually difficult waters where we are actually trying to weigh risks and benefits together in the same scales; in effect, it is basically a straightforward risk assessment rather than a risk/benefit assessment which is needed. In the other cases, the REC's judgement is indeed a subjective one; however it has the merits at least of being collective and of reflecting – if the Committee is doing its job – relevant and locally-expressed preferences as well as anyone reasonably can.

Finally the REC and the authority whom it advises are accountable for the judgements the REC makes, and as such offer a visible reference point for researchers, clinicians and patients alike. The REC is charged with making these judgements on others' behalf, and has a responsibility to do so with the protection of the research subject uppermost in its mind. In this way it is proper, if there be any leaning this way or that, for the REC to err on the side of caution, to err on the side of giving additional weight to the risks facing the research subject and of detaching itself from undue enthusiasm for expected benefits, or indeed from excessive confidence in their actually appearing. This is the REC's job, it can be done, and what is more, it can be seen to be done. Those researchers who feel obstructed by such a bias – for bias it is, and bias it should be – have an incentive as well as a duty to take whatever steps are necessary to reach their objectives by means which involve more nearly minimal risk. As for any individual potential research subjects who really wish to undergo greater risks than the REC are willing to permit, there are many alternatives to volunteering for clinical research.

The individual members of the Committee must of course construct their collective judgement not simply out of an abstract sense of the preferences and the experiences of a community which they in some way represent; they must also imaginatively project themselves into the position of the patient who may be approached to be recruited into the proposed research, research whose clinical details are before them now.   In this sense they may best represent the potential recruits by identifying themselves with them: would they themselves agree to be recruited into the trial, or (more accurately) would they agree to the recruitment of a close and dependent relative for whom they held responsibility? If the answer to this question is sincerely 'Yes', then there remains the question of whether they are satisfied with the way that the particular group of patients in question will be approached and recruited; we shall have more to say on this in the next chapter. But if the answer to the question is 'No' – if, in stark terms, they would not wish their own daughter to be recruited **in relevantly similar circumstances** to those surrounding the patient in question – it is not easy to see how they can justify permitting others to be approached.

Of course, once again this kind of reflection reminds us how personal and individual are these assessments of risk and benefit[9].   But how could it be otherwise?   For it is individual people who will be asked to take part in the research.

5.7   Minimising risk: some practical steps

Never give a sucker an even break.
(W.C. Fields)

If the view we set out in section 4.3 is right, then properly designed research can and must include safeguards to ensure that any risks involved are indeed kept to a minimum, and a number of specific items can be sought out and if necessary insisted upon by the REC, to ensure that this be done.   Of course simply following these steps will not mean that any given piece of research is thereby of only minimal risk, but at any rate some obviously needless risks can be avoided.   It is perhaps worth listing these items by way of conclusion:

- is the research design based on a genuine null hypothesis?   (is the research genuinely aimed at the apparent question?)

- are there good exclusion criteria for the recruitment of research subjects?

- are there good criteria for identifying and responding to contra-indications -

during the course of the research?

- is the researcher free from inducements (such as itemised payment per number of procedures) to perform invasive procedures which are surplus to the research subject's strict clinical requirements?

- is the consent and information procedure adequate to the features of the trial, particularly where randomisation to placebo control groups are envisaged?

- will the clinical condition of the research subjects be fully monitored before, throughout and, where necessary, after the trial period?

- is there a proper system for responding to adverse events?

- where trials are blind or double-blind, is there proper provision for immediate third-party code-breaking if it became necessary?

- are there adequate guarantees of ongoing medical support, including psychological support/counselling in appropriate cases?

Notes

1   We shall discuss this Committee in more detail in Chapter Thirteen. See also Evans, D., 'A healthcare planner's conscience', *Cambridge Quarterly of Health Care Ethics*, 3:1 (1994), pp. 108-114.

2   Nicholson, R., (ed.), *Medical Research with Children*, Oxford: Oxford University Press (1986), Chapter 5.

3   Strain, L.A. and Chappell, N.L., 'Problems and strategies: ethical concerns in survey research with the elderly', *The Gerontologist*, 22:6 (1982), p. 527.

4   Roth, L.H., Meisel, A. and Lidz, C.W., 'Tests of competency to consent to treatment', in Edwards, R.B. (ed), *Psychiatry and Ethics*, Buffalo, New York: Prometheus Books (1986), pp. 201-211; see p. 206.

5   President's Commission for the Study of Ethical Problems in Medicine and Biomedical and Behavioral Research, *IRB Guidebook*, Washington: National Institutes of Health (undated), p. 6/A/5.

6   Nicholson, *op. cit.*, pp. 106-117.

7   The scale is introduced in Rosser, R. and Kind, P., 'A scale of valuations of states of illness: is there a social consensus?', *International Journal of Epidemiology*, 7 (1978), pp. 347-58. Although it has been influential, we believe that its practical deficiencies, which lie partly in the small sample size, are eclipsed by its theoretical difficulties, not the least of which is that it requires people to assign a conjectured value to states in which they do not presently find themselves. People notoriously change their perceptions as their circumstances change. Beyond this we find the idea, of putting comparative numerical values even on states which we have experienced, basically incoherent.

8   *Guidelines*, paragraphs 3.3, 3.4.

9   It is not simply approaches to the risk/benefit balance which are individual in this sense; so too are the weightings which different people give to the various possible emphases in moral judgement, and accordingly RECs, reflecting these different weightings, can themselves differ over the moral emphasis of rights, or of beneficial outcomes, leading to the possibility that RECs may persistently but also reasonably disagree over their view of a particular protocol. See Foster, C., 'Why do research ethics committees disagree with each other?', *Journal of the Royal College of Physicians of London*, 29:4 (1995), pp. 315-8.

Chapter Six

What is this thing called 'consent'?

John Stuart Mill, Of his own free will
On half-a-pint of shandy was particularly ill
(Monty Python's Flying Circus)

6.1 The moral centrality of consent

I want you to assist me in forcing her on board the lugger;
once there I'll frighten her into marriage.
(Sydney Smith)

As we have seen, the subjects of clinical research undergo the risks of that research, and may receive no clinical benefit from doing so. If the research produces benefits, then typically these will fall to other people to enjoy. This willingness to be of service to others is one of the characteristics most admired and respected by our society, and is the basis of our determination to protect the interests of the research subject above other competing interests in clinical research. Alongside the REC's independent judgement about what risks might be permissible in any proposed medical research, the other key feature of protecting the subject's interests consists in making sure that he undertakes those risks of his own free will. The means to ensuring this lie in proper mechanisms for consent.

In a nutshell, a proper consent is a clear, open, intentional – and, we might usefully add, true – statement by the subject that he understands what he is about to do and that he freely chooses to do it. This is possible only where two conditions have been met: first his choice must be based on his possessing and understanding all the information which is relevant to making the choice; and second the choice must have been made freely, without pressure. There are of course difficulties in knowing quite how much information is 'all that is relevant' and in knowing quite what is to count as pressure, and we shall explore both of these difficulties presently. But unless it can reasonably be said that the two conditions have been met, then a proper consent has not been given.

The subject's consent is an important expression of his will, or autonomy, a notion which has enjoyed great prominence and prestige in writings about medical ethics and research ethics in recent years. Like all important ideas, it can unfortunately be over-stressed. For instance, we must be clear that no-one's autonomy can ever be absolute. Apart from the obvious point, that if people's interests conflict – and they do – then the autonomy of each must be limited by the autonomy of others, we could say also that our freedom of action as individuals is limited by our duties, responsibilities and obligations towards other people. This is not simply a complicated way of referring to their autonomy; rather it is a way of talking about our moral concerns in a language that expresses what it is to live in a society or a community. It is important that we do this when considering the research subject. A sense of gratitude and debt, towards those whose previous service as research subjects has enabled him to obtain the present array of medical treatments, can be a strong reason for someone's being willing to serve as a research subject today. It is hard for this point to be expressed in the language of individual autonomy, as it is hard for that language to express any idea of social responsibility or solidarity, matters which may crucially motivate the research subject's decision. Just as important, the notion of autonomy cannot readily give us an understanding of how it might be right to carry out medical research on those who, at the time in question, cannot meaningfully consent to being research subjects: people, for instance, who are in one or other of the special groups we mentioned above including younger children, the demented elderly, or the mentally ill or mentally impaired. We shall see that it might indeed be morally right to use such individuals as research subjects, under certain conditions. But those conditions cannot really be explained by talking about autonomy, and the consents involved will in effect be given by society rather than by the individual subject.

So we can say that in all cases the idea of consent is morally central, in that it expresses a permission to proceed, a permission that is given by the person (or, rarely, institution) most appropriate to give it. In the overwhelming majority of cases that person will be the research subject himself. And without the consent – and without a clear means to securing it, freely and fairly, as an integral part of the research design – the REC cannot approve a piece of research as being ethically appropriate. The moral centrality of consent is tied to what we could call the **procedural** centrality, in the REC's deliberations, of being satisfied that the requirements of consent are properly met.

Researchers sometimes complain that there is a kind of dual standard of consent operating between the context of ordinary clinical management and the context of clinical research, with apparently tougher requirements applying in the case of research. Of course if this is true, there are good arguments for thinking that the standards of consent in practice ought to match those in research. However if there is to remain a difference of standard, it is clear why the higher standard must apply to research: for we ordinarily assume that there is no question but that clinical practice is carried out in the express interests of the patient; by contrast, we have seen that clinical research is carried out primarily in the interests of others.

The rest of this chapter will be occupied with considering the implications of these requirements; with recognising the typical danger areas where meeting the requirements might become problematic; and with looking at possible exceptions where the requirements have to be modified.

6.2   Information and understanding

> *One [book] was* Pilgrim's Progress... *I read considerable in*
> *it now and then. The statements was interestin', but tough.*
> (Mark Twain)

Much has been said and written about the rôle of information in consent (or in 'informed consent', as it is sometimes rather redundantly called, **un**informed consent being of course no kind of consent at all). The key problems are, first, how much information is enough; second, given that absolutely complete clinical and statistical information can never realistically be conveyed to a research subject, how do we determine which is the information he needs; and third, even if we can make an appropriate choice, how can complicated technical or scientific knowledge be conveyed to a layman in terms that will mean anything to him?

These questions have sometimes been seriously presented as insuperable difficulties, making consent appear pointless or absurd – the so-called 'clinical prerogative' argument as applied to research. However, common sense tells us otherwise. \The potential research subject has a number of obvious concerns and is entitled to be reassured about them; the information he needs is therefore simply the information necessary for that reassurance. Furthermore these concerns can be expressed in straightforward, plain language – there is no earthly reason why they should not similarly be answered. The concerns are basically these:

-    why is the research being done?

-    why are you asking me to take part?

- what will I be asked to do?

- what treatment will I get if I do take part?

- will this be different from the treatment I would have got otherwise? If so, how and in what ways?

- will I get any extra or better treatment, as a result of taking part?

- can I expect to get better more quickly or more fully if I take part?

- should I expect to feel any worse for a while? Are there side effects to be expected from what will be done to me in the research?

- how will my treatment be decided? Who will decide it? Will the treatment decisions be made by my usual doctor or by someone else?

- has this sort of research been done before? Did anything ever gone wrong when these treatments were tested? Could anything go wrong now?

- what happens if something did go wrong? Am I insured? Will I be compensated?

- can I change my mind later, even if I agree to take part now? If I do change my mind, will I still get the treatment my usual doctor thinks is right for me?

These are obvious questions applying to virtually all patient-subjects of experimental research, and no doubt individual RECs and their members will think of others that are sometimes relevant in specific research contexts. The questions dictate the sort of information that is necessary for a meaningful consent. They ought to dictate also the sort of language in which the information should be given. Unfortunately all too few doctors and clinical researchers receive formal instruction in how to talk plainly and simply with patients who are invariably lay-people, and this is frequently reflected in the language of some patient consent forms and information sheets (see section 6.5) which are abrupt, terse, over-technical, otherwise incomprehensible or occasionally virtually empty. Without decent, relevant information, properly addressed in plain language to the research subject's legitimate concerns such as those presented here, meaningful consent is impossible – and the REC should withhold approval for the research to proceed unless or until the matter is put right. (The matter can be right in the first place, of course. Strikingly, in view of the commercial interests involved, we have found in our own experience of reviewing many hundreds of research protocols that many of the best current consent forms and information sheets are produced in research sponsored by the pharmaceutical industry.)

There is of course more to the question of understanding than simply whether the information is sensibly conveyed. Both the personal characteristics and the general circumstances of the research subject can have a significant effect on his ability to understand even the most clearly presented information.

Among the subject's personal characteristics, his age and level of developmental maturity are obviously important – young children cannot be expected to have the same understanding as adults. Educational problems clearly have a bearing on understanding, though significant limitations in this area are likely to be confined to those cases in which the research subject suffers from a mental impairment or other educational handicap.

The subject's circumstances are also plainly relevant. The sheer fact that patients are presently ill may be enough to impair their powers of awareness, concentration, understanding and decision-making – something we noted in considering the vulnerability of patients in section 2.2. The REC will want to take into account the likely severity of the illness of the patient group which is being contemplated: although the connection is not a strict one, more severely ill patients could frequently be expected to have more difficulties in coming to a reflective and considered judgement about whether or not they should take part in the research. Special problems can obviously arise where the patient is suffering from certain kinds of psychiatric illness.

For patients and healthy subjects alike, there are a number of factors which, whilst not bearing on the individual's powers of understanding as such (his cognitive abilities) nevertheless pose obstacles to the conveying of information to them – what we might call their apprehension rather than their comprehension of information. To take some examples, the level of an individual's educational attainment might be such that they are incompletely literate or indeed not literate at all. This obviously inhibits their understanding, although it is a difficulty that can sometimes be overcome with suitable verbal explanation. People with specific dysfunctions, such as severe impairments of sight, hearing or speech will obviously need appropriate help in gaining the information which they need. By a somewhat different token, subjects whose first language is not the language in which the research is conducted may need assistance in the form of translation.

The lesson for the researcher is not that any of these circumstances necessarily makes understanding difficult or impossible; rather it is that our ability to receive and to deal with information is a variable (and sometimes volatile) matter which is affected by many different kinds of factors. These factors must be anticipated, recognised when they are encountered, and properly taken into account. If the difficulties of understanding cannot be compensated for, then unless there are special reasons why the research can be conducted on no other subjects those subjects should not be recruited. In ordinary circumstances, the REC should satisfy itself that researchers who apply to it for ethical approval are going to take a sensitive and mature approach to judging the competence of the subjects whom they approach. Without monitoring the subject selection process, of course, the REC must – and reasonably can – assess the researcher's sensitivity from the kind of exclusion criteria she envisages and from the way she presents her information, both to the patient in terms of the wording of the consent form and information sheet, and to the Committee itself, at interview.

6.3   The recruitment of research subjects

Every time Mr Macmillan comes back from abroad Mr Butler
goes to the airport and grips him warmly by the throat.
(Harold Wilson)

Whilst many people might be broadly willing to take part in medical research if the opportunity arose, they at any rate need to be told when that opportunity does arise. Furthermore it is not likely that there will ever be enough enthusiasts, suitably ill but nonetheless volunteering unprompted to offer themselves for research purposes, to fill the places which medical research needs to be filled, in specific trials of specific treatments at specific times. It follows that most research can be carried out only if at least some of the research subjects are found from among people who are **not** clamouring for the opportunity to serve, and who have to be approached and recruited, typically whilst they are ill.

This does not mean that those who are thus recruited are acting any the less generously than are the spontaneous volunteers (indeed it could sometimes mean the reverse); neither does it mean that it is ethically dubious to recruit them. It does mean, however, that great care must be taken to ensure that the choice they make is a deliberate and reflective choice of their own free will; and this in turn means that the recruitment of research subjects is morally an extremely sensitive matter which deserves the best attention of the researcher and the REC alike. Whilst the consent of the subject to take part in research must be a continuing and on-going matter, properly facilitated by the conduct of the trial, the initial approach to research subjects is one of the points of moral focus in any research proposal, and correspondingly one of the points of focus of the REC's scrutiny.

Now as we saw in the last section, there is an important relationship between information, understanding and voluntariness. Nonetheless voluntariness consists in more than just being able to consider the necessary information – it means being free from other kinds of constraint as well. Not simply proper comprehension of the relevant information but also the opportunity to make a free and unconstrained **choice** are crucial to a proper consent. Both are clearly at stake in the process of subject recruitment. This is not simply because the initial approach must be made in a way which offers the potential recruit both the appropriate information and the appropriate circumstances in which to consider and act on it. It is also because of the special vulnerability of the research subject, something which is nowhere more relevant or important than at the time of initial approach and recruitment.

The subject's vulnerability in part consists in problems concerning just these very two considerations which we now stress as being so important: the ability to grasp and comprehend information, and the ability to make a reflective and uninhibited choice on the basis of that information, in the light of a clear conception of his or her own best interests. In the case of some patients, as we saw, simply feeling ill can make comprehension and decision-making difficult; but for all patients their freedom to choose as they would wish is always liable to be influenced by considerations of gratitude and obligation towards those whom they perceive to be the prime movers in their own recovery. Furthermore any suggestion, tacit or otherwise, of especial clinical benefit to them arising expressly out of their taking part in the research may all too easily appear to them to be an inducement to take part, an inducement moreover which might be very difficult to resist for someone who feels ill or weak and who very much wants to feel better or stronger.

In the case of healthy volunteers and controls, the comprehension and management of information may present no problems but the characteristic circumstances of many such subjects includes an element of dependency or pressure. This could be mainly economic in the case of the unemployed or members of what we might think of as in some sense 'captive' groups (medical students, pharmaceutical employees, the armed forces and so on) or it could be mainly social as in the case of family members who are recruited to serve as controls for research involving sick relatives, or who are recruited from the lists of a general practitioner on the grounds of their medical history or contacts. The economic pressure easily takes the apparent form of inducement, and is as a result something for which the REC must watch very carefully. Monetary payments for the time and expenses involved in participating can easily be coercive if they are too substantial in relation to someone's income – clearly a possibility in the case of those subsisting on state benefits or student loans. Particularly dangerous is the idea of offering higher payments for greater degrees of risk. An inducement in this context is something which inclines us to do something we would otherwise choose not to do, and if the inclination is irresistible then the inducement becomes coercion – and the resulting choice is not a genuinely free choice at all.

There is one further vulnerability which we have not yet mentioned – the vulnerability of the researcher herself. If the sponsor's need to recruit a statistically sufficiently large number of subjects is tackled by offering the researcher too large a *per capita* payment for each subject she successfully recruits, then the researcher's own ability to deal scrupulously with the problem of recruitment is itself compromised. *Per capita* payment for recruitment is even more dangerous in open-ended studies with no specified upper limit on the number of subjects to be recruited. (Similar considerations apply to payments which are made on the basis of the number of procedures carried out: such arrangements, unless carefully constrained by the protocol, represent an inducement to the researcher to put her research subjects through a particular procedure more times than is necessary, and if the procedure is at all invasive then this means more times than it is in the subject's interests to undergo.) The REC has therefore a number of good reasons for needing to know both the basis and the scale of the renumeration which a researcher expects to receive from a sponsor, and among those good reasons the question of subject recruitment is prominent. Undue pressure on the researcher to recruit will generally mean undue pressure on research subjects to take part.

In recognising these problems, the point is not that it is necessarily or even *prima facie* unethical to recruit subjects from vulnerable groups; rather it is that the different vulnerabilities of different potential subjects must be anticipated, recognised, understood and taken into consideration by both the researcher and the REC. In other words, these vulnerabilities must be actively and visibly acknowledged in the way that the subjects are identified, approached and dealt with. The REC will want to be satisfied that the research proposal has a clear strategy in this regard. Such a strategy must involve at least the following elements: first, it must justifiably assume that any general vulnerabilities of the proposed research population are inevitable, in the sense that the research could not realistically be carried out on a less vulnerable group. (We have in mind here individuals who are perhaps more mature, or less frail, or in less distress, or less weak, or less confused, or otherwise better placed to make their own decisions than the envisaged patient population. This is of course a general moral requirement of any research design, though it comes to the foreground more especially in certain specific kinds of research, such as paediatric or psychiatric research.) Second, given a justified assumption of this kind then there must be clear account taken of the likely characteristics of the patient population concerned, drawing attention to particular features such as age, dependency, any likely infirmity or impairment of the abilities of understanding and decision-making, the duration and severity of the illness concerned, the nature and expected outcomes of both the available standard clinical management and the treatment under investigation and, in this connection in particular, whether the patients in question are likely to form unrealistic expectations of what participation in the research might do for their own clinical improvement. Third, the strategy must clearly determine how potential recruits are to be identified in the first place, and must ensure that this will be done with the knowledge and cooperation of the patient's current professional carers: the REC will want to be satisfied that those presently responsible for the patient's care will have the opportunity to decide for themselves if it is clinically appropriate for a given patient to be approached, before the approach is made. Fourth, the strategy must take account of whether recruiting a given patient has implications for others, typically family members, for instance in the case where genetic research may lead to information that has a bearing on the potential health status and clinical management of other people who are not being formally recruited. The terms of the approach must neither lead to anxiety nor appear to offer unrealistic expectations of individual benefit to the subject, and they must make it unmistakably clear (and this can be formalised, as we shall see in the next section) that the subject has a genuinely free choice as to whether or not to take part.

This is of course not an exhaustive list – RECs will determine from experience of their local patient populations and the local researchers and facilities whether there are other aspects to recruitment which are important. The elements we have mentioned arise from recognising that the ideal circumstances of making free and informed choices rarely obtain when we are ill and dependent on others. If those who are already ill and dependent are to be invited to set their own interests aside to any extent, then, quite apart from the general justification (in terms of risks and benefits) for such an invitation, the invitation itself must be made in the most sensitive terms, with the door held firmly open for possible refusal. Beyond the actual selection of the potential subjects to be approached, with which we have been concerned in this section, the invitation must obviously consist in suitable information and undertakings on the part of the researcher. These are typically given substance in the Subject Information Sheet and Subject Consent Form, and we shall look at these in section 6.5.

6.4   The problem of inducement

Some circumstantial evidence is very strong, as when you find a trout in the milk.
(Henry David Thoreau)

We can be fairly certain that if Phase I drug research – the 'first time into human' studies of new therapeutic substances – depended on recruiting purely altruistic, unpaid healthy volunteer subjects (as is the case with the recruitment of blood donors in the United Kingdom) then that research would grind to a sudden halt.

There are several reasons for this. The first concerns the object of the exercise. Blood collection has a precise and dramatic objective: saving human lives imminently threatened by death. Whilst Phase I research is also in the long term meant to help us save lives or to improve their quality, the outcome is a long way off and much more uncertain. Many initially promising substances are found at Phase I to have unacceptable levels of toxicity, tolerability and bio-availability, and so their development is stopped without any lives having been saved or improved by their application. Other drugs are abandoned during later phases of development when they are found to have unsatisfactory levels of efficacy or side effects. So the immediate and direct sense of saving or improving the quality of others' lives is missing from service as a healthy volunteer in Phase I studies.

Another big difference between Phase I drug research and blood donation lies in the perceived risks of taking toxic substances whose precise effects are unknown. Whether or not the risks are real, this is clearly different from the more familiar and less threatening procedure of donating blood. Add to this the very considerable differences in inconvenience and discomfort endured by the blood donor on the one hand and the healthy Phase I volunteer on the other, and it is not surprising that some form of financial inducement to research subjects is required to keep Phase I research going.

Now it's not necessarily wrong to induce people to take minimal risks. If their health is properly protected then it might even be in their interests to volunteer (most obviously in their economic interests if their financial circumstances are difficult). Whilst up to a point they might be motivated by a concern for future patients, making their participation altruistic to that extent, there is nothing immoral as such about their participating out of pure self-interest; after all it does not, other things being equal, prejudice the interests of others. If anything their volunteering will **serve** the interests of others, even if that is somewhat beside the point as far as any given volunteer is concerned.

We accepted right at the start of this book that there are publicly accepted limits to what people should be asked to do, and we will explore this point more fully in section 6.8. So there are limits also to the inducements that may be offered to people to do what they would rather not do. We must be careful, for instance, when the extent of people's reluctance to do something is reflected in the size of the inducement necessary to effect compliance. Inordinate inducements might secure the agreement of people to engage in activities about which they have an almost inordinate reluctance. For example, whilst the offer of five pounds sterling to betray a friend would not dent our resolve to show loyalty and maintain such a relationship, the offer of a million pounds would seriously test the resolve of the best of us. We might have to admit that what makes an offer like that so obscene is precisely that it breaks down a reluctance which goes deep within us. Whilst someone's reluctance to offer herself as a healthy volunteer might not involve moral issues like these (though of course they might do in certain circumstances) some levels of inducement could still be seen as demeaning the person through showing disrespect for the deep reservations or preferences that she might have. The maxim that 'everyone has his price' is not one which commends to us those who live by it. So it is indeed a matter of moral concern to protect potential research subjects from being exploited by being offered inducements which most people would find it impossible to resist.

But now we find ourselves with a particularly tricky problem. It is that what people are capable of resisting is relative to the circumstances in which they find themselves, and the economic vulnerabilities of most healthy volunteers are self-evident. Subjects' vulnerability can't be removed: they do find themselves in these situations. Neither, as we have seen, is there any way of avoiding the reality of the remunerations offered being identified as inducements. So what can we do to minimise the risk of exploitation and lack of respect to prospective subjects?

We have already said there should be no suggestion of tying the level of payment to the level of risk. Payment should instead be made for the time given up and for the inconvenience and discomfort which the subjects must incur (we are assuming here that 'risks' concern more serious harms than these). It's a fact of life that the time of a highly-qualified, sought-after practitioner is worth more than that of an unskilled labourer in that we pay differential amounts for the time we employ them. Whilst the qualifications of research subjects are irrelevant to their usefulness in the process of research, nevertheless those of us who are fortunate enough to earn the sort of salary that buys a comfortable lifestyle by and large simply do not appear in the ranks of healthy volunteers (unless our continued employment or career prospects are threatened by our failure to 'volunteer', as might be true of employees of pharmaceutical companies). As a result, payments marginally above what might be thought to be an acceptable minimum wage would not attract the employed, though they would constitute a considerable attraction to the unemployed and student populations. (Medical students are subject to further obvious pressures to 'volunteer'.) This is an inescapable truth and it must be faced in the execution of Phase I research. The world is not an equal place and many people find themselves doing unpleasant or dangerous jobs for other people who wouldn't dream of doing those jobs, and who can afford not to. This is a fact of life, though an obvious inequality, which we accept within limits.

(No doubt we do think certain tasks would be too dangerous to invite people to perform, although the principle of 'danger money' and payment in proportion to risk is an established part of pay bargaining and employment practice. Of course what distinguishes danger money from trial participation fees is that the relationship between an employer and an employee is just not like the clinical relationship. It might be a romantic view of the clinical relationship to think of it as in some sense sacrosanct, but if so then it is a romanticism that is remarkably durable and widely held.)

At one level, then, trading on the circumstances of these groups of people to recruit them as healthy volunteers **is** exploitative, but no more so than might be the case in many areas of employment and public service. Indeed this comparison usefully draws attention to the social value of the activity. But **undue** exploitation is another matter and, though it might be difficult to measure, a good rough guide would be the offer of rewards greater than the payment for comparable jobs – that is, jobs which most of us would avoid as much as we would avoid serving as healthy volunteers. So payments for the time of healthy volunteers in line with acceptable rates of pay for unskilled work would not constitute socially unacceptable inducements when added to reasonable specific payments for inconvenient or uncomfortable procedures of various kinds, such as faecal collections and venepunctures, and for social restrictions such as bans on smoking, alcohol consumption, strenuous exercise or driving.

If this approach is suitable for healthy volunteers, what about those patients who are recruited into Phase II research? We have claimed that such patients are not straightforwardly being treated, precisely because the object of the exercise is not to help them so much as to find out what **could** help people like them. So one might well ask why they should not be offered precisely the same remuneration as healthy volunteers. Indeed during 1995 we reviewed a trial sponsored by one of the central research funding bodies in the United Kingdom which involved making payments to patient subjects in this way. This was the first offer of this sort which we had ever come across, apart from the unusual and very occasional offer to pay out-of-pocket expenses to subjects for attending hospital clinics or GP surgeries. It made us ask ourselves whether this would be a desirable trend in clinical research. On the negative side we can already anticipate the kind of cry from the heart which will come from research sponsors and researchers alike, namely that such payments will greatly increase the cost of research, to the point where much research currently performed on a shoe-string budget by enthusiastic clinicians without sponsorship would become unaffordable. But in Phase II pharmaceutical research, most projects are sponsored. What's more, only small numbers of subjects are employed and the increased expense would not be great. On the positive side the claims of fairness seem irresistible. Phase II research, quite properly, asks serious questions about whether a new medicine is going to be effective. Furthermore these subjects are being asked to put up with inconveniences and discomforts over and above those which they already have to endure as a result of their illness – their physical burden is heavier than that borne by healthy volunteers.

At Phase III it might be argued that some therapeutic benefit is more likely to be available to the subjects and the call for remuneration would not be so compelling. Certainly to pay subjects at this stage would involve very large numbers and very considerable sums of money. As the questions to be answered here more likely concern the duration of the treatment required to produce maximum benefit (or rather maximum balance of benefit), participation in the trial might be regarded as a part, though a somewhat unpredictable part, of treatment. Notice that even if we grant this much substance to the notion of 'therapeutic research' we are still left with the uncomfortable injustices suffered by patient-subjects in Phase II research without the option of receiving the financial benefits offered to subjects in Phase I. As unfairness is an ethical matter this consideration is an important one for ethical review committees.

6.5   The Subject Information Sheet and Subject Consent Form

Blurting out the complete truth is considered adorable in the
young, right up to the moment that the child says, 'Mommy,
is this the fat lady you can't stand?'
(Judith Martin)

In these two documents we have the opportunity to formalise the considerations that have been occupying us so far in this Chapter. Both should form an integral part of the research protocol and should automatically be included as part of the submission to the REC. It is surprising how often researchers fail to include either or both of these documents in their submissions, leaving the REC with the clear impression that the missing documents are not regarded as integral to the protocol. Whilst they can always be supplied for the Committee's inspection upon request, leaving them out of the initial submission hardly suggests that the researcher lays any great importance upon them – nor, perhaps, upon the substantial processes of which they are the visible and formal sign. The REC may rightly feel entitled to question such researchers thoroughly to establish to the Committee's satisfaction just how seriously the provision of information and the securing of consent are taken by those researchers.

The Information Sheet should be geared to addressing, in plain language, the questions we listed in section 6.2 – and also any others that are particularly relevant in the light of the particular piece of research in question. The onus for anticipating the subject's legitimate concerns must lie with the researcher; it should not be the subject's responsibility to labour away at extracting the information he wants, although he should of course have every opportunity to put additional questions that concern him[1]. The Committee members should ask themselves whether they are satisfied, in the case of any given information sheet, that without the benefit of specialised knowledge they would still be able to learn all that they could reasonably want to learn about the proposed research from the information provided – including answers to the specific questions we set above. There is a special rôle, perhaps, for the Committee's lay members in doing this.

The Consent Form should make it clear that the signed permissions which it contains have been given in the light of the Information Sheet. Indeed the two documents should be used in conjunction with one another. There is a good practical case for combining them into a single document, which would of course need to be duplicated so that both the researcher and the subject retain a copy. The signatures should be properly witnessed by someone who is independent of the research procedures and personnel, and who is in a position to be reasonably identified with the interests of the research subject.

Ordinarily and in the large majority of cases, these simple expedients will – when combined with a decent Information Sheet – produce a perfectly valid consent. Provided the research is ethically acceptable in all other respects, it will be able to proceed on the basis of such a consent. There are, however, problematic cases which arise when there is reasonable doubt about the competence of the research subject to consent to the research. These are the cases where in effect it is **society's** permission rather than the subject's which legitimises research on them. We shall consider these cases in the next section.

6.6   Special cases and proxy consents

To you, Baldrick, the Renaissance was just something
that happened to other people, wasn't it?
('Blackadder')

We have already listed the main specific groups of people who, by reason of special vulnerabilities which affect their ability either to understand information or to make reasoned choices regarding their own best interests, are frequently thought not competent to consent to taking part in research. However, it need not follow from this lack of competence that it is unethical to use them as research subjects. Evidently, though, they require special care and sensitivity in the way this decision is made: care and sensitivity on the part of the researcher who proposes to recruit them, on the part of the REC in deciding whether to approve the research, and care on the part of the individual (or, exceptionally, institution) that gives specific permission for the involvement of a given individual subject.

Because there are additional and special considerations which affect infants and younger children, we shall postpone discussion of these subjects until the next section. In the present section we shall be concerned chiefly with the demented elderly, the mentally or educationally impaired, and the mentally ill.

The first question for the REC to decide in assessing the ethics of proposed research on these groups concerns the necessity of using them at all: no research should be conducted on people who cannot consent on their own behalf, if it could have been just as well carried out on other people who can. The moral justification must, in this respect, rest on the scientific necessity of using such subjects. It is not difficult to see how such necessity might arise. Research on the causes and treatments of psychiatric illnesses, of certain kinds of inherited mental impairments, of organic dementia, of states of reduced consciousness, or of the chronic disabling illnesses that afflict many of the frail elderly must, sooner or later, involve the people who have the conditions in question. It is also true that other, unrelated illnesses can affect these groups of people in special ways which cannot simply be predicted or inferred from their effects on the general patient population. Obvious examples concern the possible interactions of different medications, the problems of patient compliance in adhering to multiple medication regimes or to restrictions on diet or activity or mobility, the potential difficulties of carrying out certain diagnostic or investigative procedures on adults with learning difficulties, and the particular varieties of emotional impact which might be produced by episodes of intercurrent illness upon people whose lives are already constricted to a degree and in ways which may be bewildering to them. There is clearly a case for trying to understand these phenomena more fully, and research designed to do this would evidently at some stage have to be conducted on these individuals themselves.

Any justification for research on these vulnerable groups then must begin from necessity – it must be research that could not meaningfully be performed on others. However, once the justification is apparent, then it is potentially applicable to many different kinds of research procedure, and these must then be assessed for the relative weight of risks and benefits, as must research on any other patient group. This in turn raises the question of how that assessment is to be made, and by whom. In the case of ordinarily competent subjects, the assessment is made by both the individual research subject acting on his own behalf, and the REC acting on the public's behalf. We will see in the final section of this chapter that there are moral limits to the kinds of choices which may freely or voluntarily be made by even ordinarily competent subjects, and that the REC has a public responsibility to control the range of options which research subjects can be invited to consider, even though this means effectively limiting people's freedom of choice.

If this is true of research affecting competent subjects, it is doubly true of research which concerns the specially vulnerable subjects we are now considering. In saying this, we are of course taking at face value the assumption that the vulnerability of people in these special groups consists in their being less than fully competent. Within the disciplines that study the notion of competence in decision-making (chiefly law, psychology and philosophy) different commentators sharply disagree over the truth and worth of this assumption[2]. It is undoubtedly a complicated question, and too complicated for us to do justice to it here. We can make a few relevant observations, however – for instance, concerning the importance of the notion of reduced competence. It would be morally wrong to regard people as incompetent in any regard without having good reason to view them in this way, not least because it would lead us to make unjustifiable infringements upon their freedom to make their own choices. But it seems equally morally wrong to abandon those who are actually unable to make important choices for themselves, since this leaves them open to slipping unwittingly into sequences of events that might harm them. We think that the promotion of individual freedom of choice ought to take place within the context of promoting people's best interests; indeed this is the *raison d'être* of the Research Ethics Committee as a means of public protection.

In effect, the REC's general responsibility to ordinarily competent subjects is to restrict the kinds and degrees of harm which they risk encountering from clinical research – even though individual research subjects might, for reasons personal to them, be willing to face much more significant harms. In the case of specially vulnerable subject groups, the REC's responsibility is intensified, and it is fulfilled by imposing still tighter restrictions on the harms these subject groups might face from undergoing research. Moreover, any harms beyond the minimal must be clearly tied to the prospect of benefits from the therapies being studied – in contrast to research on the general patient population, where such a link is not always necessary. To reinforce the point we can notice that in the U.K., the Department of Health's *Guidelines* handle this question by referring to the law. The Department's advice is that in the case of research subjects who cannot give their own consent to research procedures, no-one else can lawfully consent on their behalf for them to take part in any research procedure that carries a more-than-minimal risk whilst offering them no hope of direct benefit[3].

We have in this section been paying attention to the characteristics of particular **groups** of research subjects; in the process we might be in danger of overlooking the variety of different individuals within these groups. As regards competence to make decisions about clinical treatment choices, it is likely that individuals will vary greatly. For instance they will vary in the degrees to which they are afflicted by the particular kinds of condition or circumstance that we are concerned with. Moreover, competence itself is not an all-or-nothing ability; there are degrees of competence, and furthermore competence characterises our ability to do specific things. We are all more or less competent to do certain things, and more or less incompetent to do certain other things. In gauging whether or not Mr Smith is competent to consent to take part in research into the effectiveness of his psychotropic medication, we do not need to know whether he suffers from some global lack of competence (as a comatose person might); rather we want to know whether he has the specific ability to make a reasoned choice, on the basis of information which he can understand, in pursuit of a durable or stable conception of where his own interests best lie. This is generally not something that the REC can know (unless, like the case of the comatose patient, the research concerns subjects whose condition is clinically incompatible with the ability to make decisions). There might well be a reasonable doubt in Mr Smith's case. Unless the proposed research has inclusion or exclusion criteria which settle the matter from the outset, the REC can't know whether Mr Smith's participation is something he can decide for himself. In cases of reasonable doubt, then, the responsibility for gauging the patient's ability must rest with someone who is familiar with him on an individual basis. All the REC can do is to make sure that the research provides for the involvement of someone like this – someone who can identify with the interests of the particular patient, and who is independent of the interests of the research itself, in short, a proxy.

The questions that concern us in this connection are basically two: who can or should be a proxy, and what is the proxy to do? Since the answer to the first question seems to depend very much on the answer to the second, we should begin with that one. So, what is the proxy meant to be doing? The choices seem to be these: to represent the interests of the incompetent subject; to act as the 'official' voice representing a collective or social interest; to provide an alternative (or 'substituted') judgement, speaking in the place of the incompetent subject. Let's consider them all.

What is it to represent the interests of the particular patient in this context? If it's really true that we would all rather wish that the research were to be done on someone else, then the simplest account of the interests of the patient are that the research should be done on someone else, and so the proxy has an extremely simple task if all that is to be done is to represent the patient: refuse permission! A proxy who does not do this is therefore representing something rather different from this simplest version of the patient's interests. A more sophisticated version might be this: the proxy's rôle is to provide a different (or 'substituted') judgement when the one that we really want isn't available. Unfortunately problems arise for this version of what it is to represent the patient's interests; essentially we seem to lack the grounds or the evidence for any deeper or more elaborate interpretation of those interests – we seem to have to supply them ourselves. The grounds concern some sort of recognition of a collective interest in the outcome of the research. Let's assume that all relevant cases involve the possibility of benefit arising from the procedures involved; we still have the problem that those benefits come from being treated, not from taking part in a research programme. The null hypothesis doesn't allow us to work on the basis of any special benefit arising from the experimental treatment. So whilst a competent subject might be able to take a more long-term, future-directed view of his own interests, believing that he has such a significant stake in the outcome of the research that he might as well take part in it, that kind of view cannot be imputed to, nor inferred on the part of, the incompetent subject. The situation is no better if we tried to extrapolate from the alternative possible account available to the competent subject, namely that he is willing or happy to act for the sake of others: altruism can't be imputed to the incompetent subject, and claims of 'It's what he would want' can't really be taken seriously except perhaps in the case of patients whose present condition involves a (possibly post-traumatic) significant diminution of their previous state, i.e. they were previously competent and known characteristically to choose to act altruistically. Even here it's not obvious that simply representing their interests must lead one to try to extrapolate their previous moral characteristics. At any rate, since proxies can and do enter the people for whom they are responsible into some clinical research, this first account seems not to be the right one.

The second possibility was that the proxy simply acts on behalf of society's interests. This doesn't seem to be the right account either because it would generally fail to explain why proxies might refuse permission to enter suitable, though incompetent, subjects into clinical research programmes. If we assume that the research protocol's inclusion and exclusion criteria have been met, we can further assume that the incompetent subject is suitable for inclusion, and that his participation would further the objectives of the research as would the participation of any other research subject. If the research has got to the stage of being conducted, then it has passed the various review stages and we ought to assume that it is sufficiently important and sufficiently safe to have done this. Society therefore has an interest in its being carried out, and as such has an interest in the objectives being met – hence society has an interest in the participation of all suitable research subjects, all of whom must *ex hypothesi* be incompetent, since ethical justification for research on incompetent subjects depends among other things on the necessity of carrying out the research on just this group of subjects. If proxies are able to, and sometimes actually do, refuse permission for the participation of the incompetent individuals for whom they are responsible, they can't simply be representing society's interests. (We'll leave aside here the complicated and rather laboured attempts to show that society's interests are nonetheless served by procedures which encourage giving first place to the interests of the individual incompetent subject. If this is true, it is also true that the the individual proxy represents the interests of the incompetent individual first and foremost – whatever society stands to gain by putting the proxy in a position to do this.)

The third possibility was a sort of substitute for the (not available) judgement of the subject himself: that is, because we can't have the judgement we want we get a different judge. Now the question is less 'Would it be a good thing for Mr Smith if he were to enter the research programme?' and more like 'Would it be a good thing as such if Mr Smith were to enter the research programme?' – a different matter altogether. If we were right in our account of the simple representation of Mr Smith's interests, then the proxy who gives permission for the research to be carried out on Mr Smith is to some extent suppressing Mr Smith's interests, or at least the natural, simple and straightforward account of them. In permitting the participation, the proxy is setting aside the fact that it might not be the best thing for Mr Smith, and affirming that it would nevertheless be the best thing if Mr Smith goes into the research. The collective interest is being set higher than Mr Smith's individual interest – at least at its simplest level. But we could still see the proxy as representing Mr Smith's interests at a deeper level. The proxy could have the responsibility of assessing the possible harms to Mr Smith and deciding when these become too significant to be justified, either by the general benefits of the research or by the possible benefits to Mr Smith himself. In other words, the proxy represents Mr Smith's interests at the second stage, the stage at which it is possible that those interests could seriously or significantly be harmed – even though at the first stage, the stage at which we might recognise that (other things being equal) Mr Smith might well **in general** prefer not to take part in research, thwarting such a preference wouldn't in itself harm his interests significantly. On this account, the proxy who is willing to consider giving permission for Mr Smith to enter the research begins by preferring the collective or social interest, but reverts to promoting Mr Smith's interests ahead of the collective interest if his interests become threatened in any more serious way. Of the three accounts, this is the one which seems most plausible, because it is the only one of the three that can plausibly explain both the giving and the withholding of permission for Mr Smith to take part in the research.

Having established what the proxy is meant to do, we can now ask the first question which we identified above, namely who ought to act as a proxy. Most people would assume that a proxy ought to be a close relative or a friend, simply on the grounds of such a person's being relied upon to represent the interests of the incompetent subject when it really counts. Indeed probably most proxies could be found in this way. Whether, when close relatives or friends can be found, they are invariably the best people to act as proxies is another matter. To decide this, we need to think again about what the proxy is meant to do. We need to think about this anyway, in the probably unusual cases where neither close relatives or friends are available – as might be the case sometimes with subjects who are in long-term institutional care, for instance.

The 'job requirements' for a proxy include being plausibly identified with the incompetent subject's interests when it really counts (i.e. at what we called the 'second stage' above), being independent of the direct interests of the research project itself (that is to say, those who are immediately concerned with carrying it out and with promoting its results in either an intellectual or a commercial sense), and having a responsible understanding of society's needs both for successful medical research and for just and visible means of protection of its more vulnerable members. Such a person might well be a close relative or friend of the subject. However, this need not necessarily be the case. Where it was not, it might be that the person was someone generally acknowledged to exercise responsible judgement, perhaps through holding some position which was itself generally recognised to require responsible judgement. We might then think that this was the person to appoint as a proxy. But what if, in such a case, the incompetent subject does nevertheless have close relatives or friends, who simply happen not to meet all the 'job requirements' set out above? If the problem is that the relatives or friends in question have a direct academic or commercial interest in the successful completion of the research, we might think that the resulting conflict of interests could be an uncomfortable one, and that such individuals ought not to be asked to resolve the discomfort, a different proxy being found instead. On the other hand, it would seem less likely that a close relative or friend would be denied the opportunity to act as a proxy for the incompetent subject simply because they (the relative/friend) had not demonstrated a sufficient enthusiasm for representing society's legitimate interests.

This brings us to the means by which research protocols should provide for appointing proxies. Protocols envisaging the use of proxies should indicate who these are likely to be in the first instance (typically, a parent or guardian) and should include a consent form suitable for completion by the proxy. It would be highly unusual for further categories of proxy to be envisaged, and where this does happen then the REC will have to consider such proposals on their merits. Essentially the proxy must be someone who is going to be capable of representing the interests of the incompetent subject at least to the level entailed in the third perspective considered above. That is, the proxy must be sufficiently identified with the subject to be in a position to tell when the subject's interests might be significantly harmed, and must be capable of taking responsibility at that point for withholding (or possibly withdrawing) the subject's participation. (It goes without saying that the proxy must be a legally competent and responsible adult.) Ordinarily, the non-availability of a parent or legal guardian ought to be an exclusion criterion for a given incompetent subject.

In satisfying itself that proposed research on incompetent groups will involve the appointment of suitable proxies for the purposes of consent, the REC is itself implicitly involved in specifying the requirements for a suitable proxy, and is doing so partly on the basis of what options a prospective proxy would be willing to consider. For instance, no-one who was openly casual with regard to withholding permission for participation could credibly represent the incompetent subject's longer-term interests. Choosing proxies on the basis of the options they seem willing to consider is a dangerous business – and one which effectively puts the real decision in other people's hands anyway. Nevertheless, we should recognise that this does indeed happen to an extent – since a responsible researcher has to exercise some discretion in the matter of who should act as a proxy, to the extent at least of noticing and responding to any blatant conflicts of interest on the part of the persons initially identified as candidates. The REC cannot judge individual candidates for proxies, but it can and must assure itself that the proposed investigator(s) will approach the matter of appointing proxies in a responsible way.

6.7   Research on children

You can't expect a boy to be depraved
until he has been to a good school.
(H.H. Munro)

We have already recognised that children who are subjected to clinical procedures face special and additional risks simply because of the physical and psychological development which they are undergoing.   It seems clear that the problems involved in trying to secure consent from younger children also arise because the child's ability to communicate is itself still developing.   For any given child, her ability to communicate will grow with her age and experience, so her age at the time of being asked to undergo clinical research will be an important factor in estimating her ability to understand the information put to her and to make her own choices.   It will obviously affect the terms in which the information can be given to her, and researchers (who are adults) will tend to find it more difficult to convey perhaps quite complicated information in the simpler and more restricted vocabulary of younger children.   Beyond this, it is plain that different children develop their communication abilities at different rates, so a group of, say, six-year-old children could exhibit quite a variety of different levels of understanding and different levels of ability to form and communicate their own choices.

The obstacles to communication can lie on both sides of the dialogue. Not only may the child lack understanding of what is being done to her in a clinical intervention, but equally importantly the researcher may very well lack any insight into what the experiences of different clinical procedures actually mean for the child undergoing them.   The subjective experiences of pain and suffering are to some extent hidden from us when they are borne by the very young.   The fact of the distress may be obvious enough, but its meaning may not.   We have heard it suggested that younger children tend to interpret pain and illness as punishment, leading them to think that they are in some way bad[4].   Whatever the truth of this, it seems obvious that pain can be made worse by a lack of understanding.

It appears then that the general requirements for meaningful consent in research feature in all the main difficulties concerning the use specifically of children in research.   Recognising this should not, however, prevent our also recognising that some children obviously are solidly capable of giving and of withholding consent in this context.   Assuming that we could make some practical distinctions enabling us to pick out which children are able to consent on their own behalf, then we need to consider what restrictions on the involvement of children should arise in the case of those who can't consent. First, though, we should assume that in the case of children who are able to understand and decide on these matters, their own decisions should be taken seriously, and proposed research should indicate that this will happen. The rôle of parent or guardian should in such cases be essentially a confirmatory one. It might be reasonable for a parent or guardian to override a child's willingness to take part in research which the competent adult believes to be against the child's interest: but there should be no corresponding opportunity for the parent or guardian to override the capable child's refusal. The REC should satisfy itself firmly on this point.

This approach, we think, can work well enough in the case of children who are capable of giving and withholding permission on their own account. Things are much more difficult in the case of children who lack that capability. Interestingly, the somewhat troublesome distinction between therapeutic and non-therapeutic research may help us here; indeed the law in England and Wales probably relies on this being true, as we shall see. Having called the simplest version of that distinction into question, we think that it can nonetheless stand in these terms: there is a clear difference between, on the one hand, research in which it is intended that all shall receive a treatment from which they could in principle benefit (at least so far as is known), and on the other hand research in which there is no such possibility (such as the study of investigational procedures concerning basically untreatable conditions like muscular dystrophy). Let's first confine our attention to 'therapeutic' research in the sense in which we have now defined it. The question immediately arises as to whether the mere possibility of benefit justifies the use of non-competent children or infants in research. Such a justification would obviously depend, first, on the value and importance of the research (for instance, children in general must benefit, or the research must be 'worthwhile' in the colloquially utilitarian terms of the British Paediatric Association's current guidelines); and, second, on the necessity of the research in the present case. The nature of this necessity must be spelled out a little. In essence, the research must be of a kind which simply could not be conducted on any other groups than on children such as those in question. This form of necessity is a perfectly practical requirement, for the very reasons attaching to the problems of the harms which are specific to these groups: there are some (mainly developmental or growth) processes exhibited in children which are just not found in adults; and the results of much pharmacological research on adults can't be extrapolated to children, who metabolise many substances differently (leading in paediatric medicine to the routine use of drugs which are not licensed for the relevant indications in children).

It seems to us that, where the relevant benefits are not outweighed by possible harms to the child subjects themselves (on which tricky matter see Chapter

Five), paediatric research which is both necessary and worthwhile in the senses defined here can be justified in such terms, even on children and infants who cannot play a full rôle in the consent process. The REC's task is therefore to be satisfied that these two requirements are met in proposed research on children, and to be satisfied also that the relevant proxy consent arrangements are satisfactory. However, whilst this justification may work when there are real benefits potentially available to the subjects themselves, the same justification is obviously just not available in the case of research from which the subjects cannot themselves benefit. The law in England and Wales awaits a test case, but the clear advice of the Department of Health is that it is unlikely that anyone could give a lawful consent on behalf of a child for that child to be entered into research from which she could expect no benefit, and which carried any risk above the absolute minimum. (The 'glue ear' study illustrates just such a combination of features, and was rejected by the REC for precisely that reason.)

We have rather taken it for granted that in practical terms it is possible to pick out which children are capable of being meaningfully involved in the consent process. We do think that this is true, but the relevant practicalities are primarily a matter of the experience and sensitivity of the researcher, something that cannot be codified in a protocol and something moreover which the REC will have to judge for itself in the case of each individual applicant (something which cannot seriously be attempted without interviewing the researcher). Part of the reason for this is that 'competence' as a phenomenon is not a single, all-or-nothing attribute magically gained in the moment of reaching the age of legal majority. None of us is competent at everything, and competence is a specific idea tied to particular skills and tasks, rather than being a global, indivisible feature of personality. Given that we all have ranges of specific competences, which ones do children develop first? No general answer to this can be given. Neither can we say which specific competences are necessary precursors or contributors to the ability to make these sorts of decisions. In the abstract we are forced to say rather general things, such as that the child will need to understand reasonably sophisticated ideas about bodily causes and effects, and that she will need to be able to form a picture of her own future interests beyond simply the short-term ones of avoiding immediate discomfort. Again, no-one can say in the abstract how much of this sort of understanding is necessary, or where lies the cut-off point beyond which the child has just enough of the right sort of understanding. A good course for a researcher to follow is to credit the child with the benefit of any doubt: where a child displays evidence of a persistent and above all **reasoned** unwillingness to undergo a particular research procedure, then we doubt whether it would be wise or proper for a researcher to disregard that unwillingness, even were the child's parents inclined to override it.

6.8   Limits to consent

If any demonstrator lays down in front of my car,
it'll be the last car he ever lays down in front of.
(George C. Wallace)

So much is made of the idea of consent in debates on health care ethics that one could sometimes be forgiven for thinking that little else mattered, morally speaking. But a moment's thought shows us that, if a valid consent were the only moral prerequisite for research, then RECs could simply confine their attention to a study of the patient information sheet and consent form. So long as these accurately and faithfully reflected the content of the research protocol – so long, that is, that anyone going into the research would do so with his eyes open – then the requirements of consent would be satisfied, and that would be that. The only additional stipulations would concern the consenting capabilities of the research subjects, and we have seen how these can be dealt with. Yet it is obvious that an REC which looked no further than this would have done only half the job, since an equally crucial part of its work, namely assessing the balance of risks and benefits which the research subjects could expect to face, would be ignored completely. And in our view, it is no answer to this simply to claim that the decision as to what is an acceptable risk/benefit balance is purely the business of the research subject. For the REC system is based on the belief that there is a public responsibility to protect individual research subjects from being invited to undergo inappropriate risks – to protect them, in other words, from being invited to neglect their own best interests.

It is true that the ultra-libertarian can object to this belief, arguing that people must be free to undergo whatsoever risks they choose. The requirement for valid consent, on such a view, is indeed the supreme moral protection of the individual, and by the same token it is the only one that is necessary or indeed tolerable. In disagreeing with this extreme libertarian view, we are partly drawing attention to the practical limitations on consent. The sheer vulnerability of many typical research subjects can defeat the very freedom of choice which the libertarian presumes must obtain. Just as importantly, society has a stake in the character of clinical research, since like all organised transactions among individuals, the way in which clinical research is conducted contributes to the way in which society conducts its affairs more generally. Society's interests are protected and developed by the regulation of all kinds of public transactions, from the regulation of the professions to the laws on consumer protection and public health. Individuals can operate freely only within the rules of these transactions, and the rules are there partly to protect the individuals concerned, but also to protect the public interest. Only the arch-libertarian will discount the idea of social or collective interests, but then the arch-libertarian has a radically different conception of what 'the good society' looks like. This is not the place to debate the merits of different conceptions of 'the good society': ethical review of clinical research takes place within societies which broadly recognise the idea of the public good.

The limits on what an individual can consent to are therefore set by two kinds of considerations, namely the public interest and also the interests of the individual: moreover, the interests of the individual are partly specified by society. This can be seen in instances as diverse as the compulsory wearing of car safety belts, the regulation of the sale and distribution of medicines, the unlawfulness of assisting someone else's suicide even at that person's request, the obscenity laws and the prohibition of certain kinds of self-harm and of certain forms of sexual expression. These things are regulated in large part to protect people from the consequences of their own decisions; to this extent modern liberal societies are paternalist under the skin, and the research ethics committee system is another expression of this paternalism. Individuals can have good and bad reasons, private to themselves, for being willing to take risks that most of us would find unacceptable. Of course, both selfless heroism on the one hand and despairing, Devil-take-all gestures on the other do have their place in private life, but neither is the sort of thing that society can invite, in cold blood and on paper: taking part in clinical research must never be the health-care equivalent of either 'going down with the ship' or joining the French Foreign Legion. Hence it is necessary that an individual's participation in clinical research must be something that he has consented to, on the basis of an invitation that society, through the deliberations of the REC, considers it is appropriate to put to him. If either party – the REC or the individual subject – is unhappy, then that participation should not come about.

Notes

1   For a clear summary of what is involved in writing a properly usable information sheet, together with a convincing account of why such advice is still necessary, see Alderson, P., *Spreading the Word on Research*, London: Consumers for Ethics in Research/North East Thames Regional Health Authority (1994).

2   Contrast the view of competent choice offered in March, J.G., 'Bounded rationality, ambiguity and the engineering of choice', in Bell, D.E., Raiffa, H. and Tversky, A. (eds), *Decision Making; Descriptive, Normative and Prescriptive Interactions*, Cambridge: Cambridge University Press (1988), pp. 33-57, with the view offered in Buchanan, A.E. and Brock, D.W., *Deciding for Others: the Ethics of Surrogate Decision Making*, Cambridge: Cambridge University Press (1989). The contrast is explored in Pickering, N., 'Deciding ways' (unpublished manuscript, available upon application to the authors of this volume).

3   Department of Health, *Local Research Ethics Committees*, London: Department of Health (1991), para. 4.4.

4   We are grateful to Louise de Raeve for drawing this suggestion to our attention.

Chapter Seven

The value of a committee – expertise, representation and accountability

7.1   The rôle of expert knowledge

One of the key requirements of good ethical review is that it be properly informed.   The REC must have an understanding of the scientific importance and validity of the submitted protocols, no matter how prestigious the 'central' ethical approval which a protocol may already have received.   This understanding is essential in order to appreciate the benefits that are possible from the research.   On the side of risks, the REC must be able to assess the pharmacology of drugs or the clinical appropriateness of dressings, surgical techniques, or sociological and psychological questionnaires, and to discern whether there are any special factors in the local study population that will influence how the proposed procedures will be applied or tolerated.   Again, the REC is particularly well placed to know of other concurrent or recent local research in the same or related clinical areas, and must apply this knowledge to the question of whether particular study populations are being over-researched, whether there is any conflict among different proposed medications or treatments, and so on.   It seems to follow straightforwardly from this that the REC should be composed of as many expert and experienced clinicians and scientific researchers as possible.

On the other hand, one of the key requirements of ethical review is that it be independent of the research interests in question, able to stand at a sufficient distance from the research is to be able to examine the interests of the prospective and actual research subjects, free from the influence of such considerations as how interesting or prestigious or important the proposed research might be. Above all other interests, the REC must protect and promote the interests of the research subject, who will be perhaps ill, certainly vulnerable, and frequently lacking in knowledge or understanding or access to information. To do this job properly a committee needs to identify with, and stand in the shoes of, the prospective research subject, whilst remaining free to make the necessary and sometimes vigorous enquiries - enquiries which sometimes may seem inhibited by professional and inter-professional responsibilities within the clinical community itself. It seems to follow from this that the REC should be composed of as many concerned laymen and women as possible!

Of course the truth is that the REC needs both lay and professional clinical input, a fact well recognised in the United Kingdom Department of Health's *Guidelines*. Quite how best to secure this input is perhaps less clear. In particular, should expertise be one of the central guiding considerations in the matter of REC membership? In practical reasoning it is often useful to consider analogies with other situations with which we are familiar. Given the adjudicatory rôle of the REC, one analogy that comes to mind is that of the jury in legal processes. Here, the adjudicatory body is essentially a lay panel, advised and to some extent directed in its deliberations by expert professionals, but nonetheless - and within certain limits - free to come to its own decision. It is true that the decisions of a jury can be overturned on appeal, and that the appeal is made to higher courts from which lay opinion and judgement is effectively absent; and it is also true that the ordinary operation of the jury system relies on the quality of the information and professional advice given; but at any rate the system has a long history and enjoys a generally accepted and established position at the heart of many judicial processes. It is at least possible, then, that the jury system provides us with a model for ethical, as distinct from legal, review. (In the next chapter we will see that the judicial analogy helps us to explore the question of independence; here our concern is with expertise.)

In the legal situation, the essential factual knowledge is provided by witnesses, and the procedural knowledge by the court's administrative and judicial officials. Witnesses inform and lawyers and judges advise (and when necessary instruct) the jury as to the allowable and relevant considerations, the pertinent material facts and their weight, and the strength and testability of evidence. In short, the rôle of expert knowledge is fulfilled in the process of legal review by making the relevant professionals available to the lay adjudicators. If the disadvantages of an essentially lay REC concern such a committee's lack of expert knowledge, this deficiency could evidently be made up for by a panel of professional witnesses and advisers, leaving the advantages of independence completely intact.

However, there is more to an effective jury system than this. The lay jurors do not take part in the process of setting out or cross-examining of evidence. For this they must rely on the expert professionals, namely the respective Counsels and the presiding Judge, who between them provide a properly adjudicated adversarial system of enquiry. This system makes sure that the relevant evidence is produced, and that it is subjected to searching enquiry of a kind that is possible only on the part of expert and experienced professionals. The jury's verdict is certainly non-expert: but it is also able to be a responsible one, precisely (and only) because the necessary enquiries have been conducted on the jury's behalf by the people competent to do it. By contrast the all-lay REC as we have so far described it would have to rely on the hope that, without benefit of expertise in medicine, nursing, pharmacy, surgery or any of the other relevant disciplines, they will still be able to penetrate the scientific case presented by the applicant before them – an applicant who may be presumed to be expert – by means of the questions that happen to occur to them. We need only to set out this hope clearly in order to see it as forlorn. Therefore to complete the analogy between the legal jury and the all-lay REC we would have to build in a system of expert inquisition, possibly an adversarial one under impartial adjudication, to facilitate the Committee's verdicts.

Of course the cost of such a system is already a huge burden in the legal arena, where in a certain sense much more is typically at stake in the decisions taken there than is usually at stake in the ethical review of research. If we continue to support the expense of the legal system then that is for other, partly historical and partly evaluative reasons which we cannot realistically transfer to the process of ethical review, itself already badly underfunded and under-resourced. If we wanted to kill ethical review stone dead, there are few simpler ways of doing so than to force it into an economically ruinous mould. Nonetheless there are lessons to be drawn from the jury analogy. We should not allow ourselves to think, for instance, that only professionals can take significant decisions in matters concerning their profession: if this is true in law, it is certainly true in the proper conduct of medical research. No-one can plausibly argue that the need for expert knowledge should exclude lay involvement in the process of ethical review. Neither should we allow ourselves to think that the lay involvement must be confined to a small minority simply as a result of the need for expert knowledge. The economic considerations are another matter and must be inspected separately, but the need for expert knowledge is compatible with an essentially lay decision-making process.

Precisely what the balance should be between the lay and the professional constituencies is a question that must reflect the distinct problem of representativeness, a problem we shall acknowledge in section 7.4. However, once we have admitted the principle of harmonising expert knowledge with lay decision-making, we can consider ways of making that knowledge available to the REC without prejudging the subsequent question of the lay/professional balance of membership.

One obvious problem for even an all-professional committee is that not all disciplines and sub-disciplines can be represented in a group of workable size: unless the number of members is to be unmanageably large, some protocols will necessitate drawing on expert knowledge not possessed by the committee. So even an all-professional committee needs some mechanism for getting access to specialist clinical and scientific information and advice on some aspects of some research proposals. The UK Department of Health's *Guidelines* envisage and encourage the use of expert advisors from the various clinical specialties, who would be consulted when the need arose[1]. The *Guidelines* do not go into detail, so it is worth our thinking about how the mechanism might work. Assuming an agreed means of identifying when and which area of expertise was needed, the relevant protocol could be sent to the professional concerned in advance of a committee meeting. That person could then be invited to attend the meeting for the relevant agenda item, addressing the members and responding to their questions. Ideally, and if appropriate, he or she might also take part in the interviewing of the research proposer, and subsequently contribute to the committee's discussion of the interview. However, beyond the giving of clear and unequivocal advice, which the REC should obviously take very seriously, he or she should not formally have a rôle in the decision itself, for reasons considered in the next section. Equally, the expert advisor ought not to be a periodic, nominal member of the REC representing his/her discipline. The identity of the committee is important, and there is no need for this identity to be blurred by the taking of occasional expert opinion, as the jury analogy clearly shows.

7.2   The Department of Health's *Guidelines* on representation

> *Really, if the lower orders don't set us a good*
> *example, what on earth is the use of them?*
> (Oscar Wilde)

It is worth quoting the *Guidelines'* advice on the question of representation. Paragraph 2.6 notes that:

> Despite being drawn from groups identified with particular
> interests or responsibilities in connection with health issues,

> LREC [Local Research Ethics Committee] members are not in
> any way the representatives of those groups. They are appointed
> in their own right, to participate in the work of the LREC as
> individuals of sound judgement and relevant experience.

This emphasis on the individual character of the REC member is interesting. It may rest on an assumption that the moral concerns which should mobilise the REC's work do not come from particular professional or other interested groups but rather from society as a whole, of which all mature and responsible citizens are members. If this is the assumption, it seems a good one. 'Sound judgement' in matters of morals comes from experience of living in society as a whole, and not from working in any particular profession. This is not to deny the importance of specialist professional knowledge, nor indeed to deny its moral relevance, as we saw in the previous section; 'relevant experience' clearly can include clinical experience. But it is to insist that the moral conclusions which should be drawn in the light of specialist clinical information are nonetheless drawn on the basis of wider concerns – concerns which we are qualified to promote, if we are qualified at all, simply by living responsible lives. In this sense, the experiences of the lay members of a committee are as important as those of the clinicians, and the *Guidelines'* following paragraph advises that at least one of the lay members should be 'unconnected professionally with health care and be neither an employee nor adviser of any NHS [National Health Service] body'[2].

There are other aspects to this emphasis on individuals. One concerns the importance of individual members' freedom from having simply to champion the prior and already laid-down concerns of some constituency of professional opinion, which would of course reduce the member to being little more than a delegate with a mandate. Another crucial dimension of this concerns the way that the Committee functions together as a group. Moral discussion flourishes best in a situation of trust, where contributors to the discussion can speak freely, without inhibition, and without confining themselves to prepared positions. For this to happen the members of the REC need to get to know one another over a period of time and to have the opportunity to develop a sense of respect for each other. This can happen in a committee made up of given individuals, in a way in which it cannot happen in a committee made up merely of delegates, whose individual identity is unimportant. For this reason, although the *Guidelines* do not say so, it is important that the membership of the Committee be so far as possible a settled one, in which the same individuals meet regularly and establish genuinely personal working relations. The habit of sending others to deputise should be actively discouraged; deputies too readily become delegates. What's more, relying on deputies diminishes one's own rôle in a discussion (as well as, obviously, the rôle of the deputy herself) to something much more like the mere representation of a position.

Beyond this, it also disrupts the development of genuinely personal working relations.

7.3 Traditional problems of representation

The man who is denied the opportunity of taking decisions of importance
begins to regard as important the decisions he is allowed to take.
(C. Northcote Parkinson)

Solving the above problem of independence does not of itself guarantee effective ethical review, given that effective ethical review is there first and foremost to protect the interests of the research subject. All-professional committees from within a given establishment, mutually reviewing each others' research proposals, would be weak because they embodied interests which were too close to the interests of those pursuing or conducting any given piece of research, and as such they could not credibly be seen to promote the interests of those on whom the research was to be carried out. But one could be independent of the conduct of research and yet still fail to stand up sufficiently for the research subject, for instance because one took an overly utilitarian view of the interests of society. That view might lead one to regard medical research as a good to be promoted in a dispassionate manner; on such a view it would still be morally important to take a detached and critical look at the value of the research, independently of the interests of those conducting it, but it might well seem morally permissible or even obligatory to subordinate the interests of a few individual research subjects to the greater good of the community, particularly if the 'greater good' in question concerned obviously important medical advances, or if the harms which faced the research subjects seemed to be not so very serious. Fairly obviously, we would not want our ethical review to be conducted by people who took this view. What seems to be lacking is any sense of their identification with the interests of the ordinary research subject. Of all the members of the REC it is to the lay members that the public first looks to provide this sense of identification.

If we look again at some of the traditional patterns of membership of RECs – at any rate in Britain – we might at first think we can pick out this lack of identification in the kind of lay members habitually appointed to the Committee. There is a strong British tradition of selecting lay contributors to public bodies from among a rather narrow section of society, typically middle- or upper-middle class, and characteristically patrician in outlook. This was true of the lay membership of RECs until relatively recently, widely expected to be drawn from a stock repertoire of stalwarts, typically professionals or retired professionals. Such people would be used to assessing and judging the behaviour and ideas of others. The senior medical professionals who historically dominated RECs would have found it easier to accept the involvement of lay men and women in their professional deliberations if the laity in question were socially accomplished, if they understood and were sympathetic to the perspective of medical authority, and if they were educated but nonetheless deferential on matters outside their own expertise, as they in turn expected deference from others. The 'tokenism' of the resultant situation is obvious; moreover, the lay members of the Committee, to the extent that they represented anybody, represented that section of British society which was least likely to appear in the research subject population[3].

Tokenism in the sense described here seems self-evidently a bad thing. However, whether a lack of identification with socially more typical research subjects is necessarily harmful is less clear. First, it is plausible to suppose that the educational advantages traditionally enjoyed by the 'patrician' section of society might – if exercised without fear, favour or inappropriate deference to medicine's authority – work to the advantage of effective ethical review. But perhaps these educational advantages have been largely dispelled in recent years; certainly educated and intelligent lay men and women can be found from all social strata. A more serious reason to doubt whether the key to effective review necessarily lies in a more representative laity is that the idea of representativeness is itself somewhat limited when a small committee of twelve or so persons is meant to reflect the complexity and variety of modern industrial society. Clearly, two or three lay members cannot between them even hope to represent the variety of research subjects with which the Committee will be concerned: the variables include at least socio-economic background, educational attainment, age, gender, ethnic background, occupational rôle, social rôle and – pretty importantly – health status. If these variables are important – and presumably they are – then clearly no Committee can even begin to approach the reflection of a cross-section of the population whose interests they nominally represent.

The nearest approach to such a cross-section would be achieved by selecting an all-layperson Committee according to tightly defined criteria. The obvious price to be paid for this strengthened representativeness is an immediate, and perhaps total, loss of the professional expertise necessary for the evaluation of the research proposals coming before the REC: scarcely progress towards effective ethical review. We can recall that there is something to be said in reply to this objection, in that a precedent for an essentially lay adjudication process exists in the legal jury system, but we have already considered and dismissed this idea on grounds of cost and ineffectiveness, in section 7.1. However it might be argued that as an approach to proper representation, even this all-laity REC was insufficiently radical, since the really interesting cross-section of society (and the one that we most ought to want in this context) is not a general cross-section but a specific one of the actual patient population; hence the REC should be composed of a representative selection of current and former patients and research subjects!

There is indeed something to be said for this radical idea: the proposers of research would certainly have their minds concentrated on the problems of maximally protecting the interests of the research subjects, if they were to be at all confident of obtaining ethical approval for their projects. However, at this point we should recall the limitations on the consent process which we considered in section 6.8 above. It is possible that at any rate current and former research subjects have, by their own proven willingness to take part in medical research, adopted a sympathetic attitude to it which might in their own cases have led them to consent to things which were not in their own best interests – were it not for the restraining hand of the ethical review process. We have already seen that a large part of the REC's work consists in making judgements about what people ought to be permitted to consent to; it is not obvious that those judgements can be made with sufficient detachment and independence by people who have already allied themselves to the general project of medical research, even in the capacity of willing subjects. Perhaps researchers' trepidations about the all-ex-subject committee would turn out to be surprisingly misplaced. For obviously similar and corresponding reasons, the same might be true of a Committee composed entirely of patients and ex-patients who had not, as a matter of fact, been involved in research. Such a Committee would appear to satisfy the requirement of independence in a way in which the ex-research subject Committee could not, but nevertheless, current and former patients face the familiar vulnerabilities of being either in present need of what the medical staff can offer them, or in debt for what has already been done. Again it is, to say the least, unclear that such a Committee would even begin to provide an effective critical scrutiny of the moral acceptability of proposed research.

We have now encountered two important limitations on the idea of representation. The first is a practical limitation: twelve or fewer individuals simply cannot in any meaningful sense reflect a cross-section of modern society or of the patient population they are there to protect. The second is ultimately a moral limitation: a case can be made for preferring this or that group of people or group of rôles in the REC of one's choice, but such a preference reflects one's own view of how best to achieve the protection of the interests of the research subject; and any view on this question which is not simply confined to putting the responsibility entirely on the subject's own decision-making is to that extent a paternalist view. It is a basic assumption of ethical review as we are describing and exploring it in this book that the interests of the research subject must be to some extent defined and protected by other people. Our preferred choice of REC committee members is therefore simply a question of whom we most trust to define and protect those interests. This is a moral question, first and last.

7.4   The constitution of the Committee

The phrase 'properly constituted' is a familiar one from most contexts where
public decisions have to be taken in a formal way by a group of people who
have been instructed, or who claim authority, to do so.   It reflects our concern
that those decisions should themselves have the authority they will need if they
are to be effective.   This means that they must be able to withstand scrutiny and
reasonable challenges, both procedural and on occasion legal.   To do this they
must have been taken in good faith, according to established and recognised
procedures, by a body of people properly authorised and qualified to take them.
The authorisation should itself be tied to, among other things, the recognised
competence of that group of people to take the decisions.   The sentiment that
'Justice must be done and be seen to be done' applies to the idea of proper
constitution of the REC.   When the protection of the interests of vulnerable
subjects of medical research is at stake, we have a powerful reason for making
sure that the REC's decisions are properly taken and will command respect and
confidence in those whom they affect – researcher and research subject alike.

7.4.1   Relationships with commissioning authorities

In Britain, the REC is an advisory committee to the local Health Authority
(usually though not necessarily at the level known as the District).   The
Health Authority sets up the REC with the specific job of advising on
whether proposed research, intended to be carried out within the
geographical area of that Health Authority, is ethically appropriate.
However as the Department of Health's 1991 *Guidelines* make clear, the
REC is not an arm of management of the Health Authority[4].   The REC is
meant to be offering independent advice, and independence in this context
means that the REC must be free from the managerial and economic
considerations which the Health Authority itself is obliged to consider.
(Clearly, such considerations must be kept scrupulously apart from the
central question of whether or not any proposed research is contrary to the
interests of the subjects who might be enrolled in it, something we shall
stress in section 8.2.)   The Constitution of the REC must make this
relationship with the commissioning Authority clear, as an integral part of
stating the REC's purpose.

In this connection, the Constitution should make clear the REC's actual powers, since they are not the executive powers held by the Health Authority itself. In Britain, the REC has the power **to provide, to withhold or when necessary to withdraw ethical approval** in connection with any piece of proposed research placed before it. This is the character and the scope of the advice which it supplies to the commissioning Authority, and the Authority is entitled, and ordinarily can be expected, to take executive action on the basis of that advice. The REC's Constitution should state these powers, again as an integral part of defining the Committee's function.

The Constitution then is a statement of the REC's nature, rôle, responsibilities and relations with the Authority whom it advises. The details of the Constitution set out the way in which its decisions will be considered and taken, as we shall see below. Finally the Constitution should be a public document, so that the reassurances which it should embody will be properly available.

7.4.2   Composition, membership and meetings

We have already discussed the important ideas of expertise and representation on the Committee and in the next chapter we will look more closely at a further key requirement of an REC, namely its independence. General provisions for ensuring these features should be reflected in the Constitution. In particular, the rôle of the lay members should be made clear. In Britain the Department of Health *Guidelines* recommend that either the chairman or vice-chairman should be a lay member, and unless there are compelling reasons to the contrary, we believe this recommendation should be followed[5]. The independent character of ethical review is at least signalled by giving some formal prominence to the lay membership, and the Constitution should make clear whether this recommendation is being followed. Once the features of a generally accepted framework for membership have been established, the framework should be expressed in the Constitution. An example of such a framework is one which ensures that the major relevant kinds of expertise are represented on the Committee, yet which avoids the representation of sectional interests. Thus for instance it is important to have the input of pharmacological or nursing expertise, but not necessarily important – at least from the point of view of ethical review as such – to have representatives of the Health Authority's pharmaceutical or nursing administration. Whilst administrative experience is important when studying management and resource questions, these are not primarily the questions which the REC is asked to consider. The Constitution can make clear whether or not the Committee's clinical expertise is tied to professional administrative functions. Similarly, whether or not the lay members ought to represent patient consultative or representative bodies (Community Health Councils in Britain) or indeed for that matter represent the commissioning authority itself (District Health Authorities in Britain) is a question that ought first to be settled, and then to be effectively recorded in the REC's Constitution.

The traditional rules of meetings obviously require the Constitution to specify the number of members the Committee is to have, and the Department of Health *Guidelines* advise that between eight and twelve is appropriate[6]. It is usual for the Constitution to specify the normal term of appointment of members and of Officers (generally the Chairman and vice-Chairman), the circumstances within which members must be appointed and Officers elected, and the mechanisms by which members or Officers may be removed if necessary. The Constitution should also record the number of members whose presence is required to make any meeting quorate, and there are good reasons for requiring the quorum to include the presence of certain rôles, such as a nurse, a general practitioner, a pharmacist and a lay member.

A further public indication of the character of the REC's work is the frequency of its meetings. Whilst this will obviously reflect the Committee's workload, and workloads vary among different health commissioning authorities, the workload for a given Committee will be reasonably predictable. The public, and particularly the patient/research subject population, are entitled to know whether their REC has sufficient meeting time to give proper consideration to the research protocols before it and to process them effectively, and hence the Constitution should specify the frequency of the Committee's meetings. In combination with the Annual Report detailing the actual workload (discussed in the next section), this will give the public some of the vital information it needs in order to judge whether the REC is properly able to fulfil its protective function. The question of whether meetings should be held in public or in private is difficult, and we will consider it in more detail below. Since it is at best arguable whether this question, unlike the frequency of meetings, strictly affects the ability of the REC to fulfil its function, it is doubtful whether the Constitution needs to refer to this point.

Like all other matters in the Constitution, questions of composition, membership and meetings should be open to periodic review to see whether the present arrangements are the best under the circumstances. The Constitution should in any case, under the traditional rules of meetings, allow for amendments, and should specify the requirements which must be met for amendments properly to be made.

7.5   The Annual Report

The chapter on the Fall of the Rupee you may omit. It is somewhat too sensational.
(Oscar Wilde)

The production of a Report is a traditional way of recording to what extent, and by what means, responsibilities have been carried out. The REC has an obvious responsibility to the commissioning health Authority, and an Annual Report can record in summary form how the responsibility has been met. The Department of Health's *Guidelines* in fact recommend that the Annual Report should be sent to all the National Health Service bodies who are advised by the REC – this means, in addition to the Health Authority, the various hospitals, trusts, general practices, and perhaps medical and nursing schools who may have been involved in carrying out research which the REC considered. These bodies have a clear clinical and managerial interest in knowing what research has been submitted to the REC, and how the REC judged it and on what grounds. Beyond this, the *Guidelines* envisage that the Annual Report should be available for public inspection. It could well be argued that the public has a corresponding interest in knowing precisely this information.

Difficulties arise here. It seems obviously right that the Report should be available for public inspection, since after all it is ultimately the public, from whom research subjects are recruited, whom the REC exists to protect. Without compelling reasons to the contrary – and we envisage none – the public should certainly be able to examine the activities of the REC and consider whether it has been properly able to carry out its protective function. The Annual Report provides an obvious mechanism by which this can happen. However, what sort of information could give the public the reassurance that they should reasonably want? Unlike the proceedings of Parliament, public enquiries or (in most cases) the Courts, the proceedings of the REC are not themselves conducted in public. We shall consider in the final section of this chapter whether in fact they should be. But at any rate they are not public proceedings now. Indeed the Department of Health's *Guidelines* envisage (for reasons which we will consider) that REC meetings will normally be private and the minutes taken will be confidential to the committee. Accordingly there is a gap, perhaps a substantial one, between the sort of information that will appear in confidential minutes, and the sort of information that can appear in a public Report. Presumably this is why the amount of information which the *Guidelines* regard as necessary for the Annual Report, is rather limited: 'the names of Committee members, the number of meetings held and a list of proposals considered (including whether they were approved, approved after amendment, rejected or withdrawn)...'[7]. Is this amount of information enough for the public to know whether they can have confidence in how the protective function of the REC has been carried out?

The listed information is certainly necessary. That is to say, on the basis of at any rate some of this information one could certainly know if one ought not to have confidence in how the REC does its job: if the number of meetings is clearly insufficient to consider the number of protocols, or if all protocols are straightfowardly approved, year after year, without amendments ever being required, then the public can reasonably conclude that the review is not effective. On the other hand, the information really does not seem sufficient. For instance, simply giving the names of committee members without any indication as to their rôles or professional backgrounds will leave it an open possibility that the committee be composed entirely of consultant doctors from the local general hospital. No such committee would nowadays be thought proper, and the public is entitled to know that their REC has a balanced membership with an appropriate range of expertise and an appropriate degree of independence. Again, what counts as a 'list' of proposals considered? The *Guidelines* do not advise as to whether this means simply the title of a particular study, which will mean little or nothing to most members of the public – even to those relatively few who would take the trouble to find and inspect the Annual Report itself – or whether it means in addition the name of the sponsor and of the proposed investigator, which would at least enable the public to observe whether a given sponsor or investigator engages in substantial quantities of research, and whether they generally receive approval or are sometimes (or indeed regularly) required to modify or even withdraw research proposals. No doubt some will take the view that the public is not helped by this kind of information, but the case needs to be made. There seems no obvious reason why the REC's independent and impartial functioning should not be assessed by seeing how it adjudicates with respect to the individuals and companies concerned, as well as with respect to the different sorts of study title.

Having gone as far as this, we might further ask whether the general reasons for requiring amendment or for rejection should not be noted in the Report. Now there are doubtless some limits that would have to be placed on this, in that it is reasonable for researchers and for sponsors to enjoy a certain amount of protection of commercial and scientific confidentiality; nonetheless there is still a case in favour of general information of this kind, arising from the public's reasonable need to know the sorts of considerations that govern the Committee's thinking and judgement. If, for example, amendments are requested and agreed by the researcher, it is hard to see why the reasons for the amendment should not be a matter of public record, counting moreover to the credit of both Committee and researcher; again, if research is rejected in view of requests for appropriate amendments which are put forward by the REC but are – perhaps repeatedly – unmet, it is not obvious why the public should not know this. At the end of the day clinical research is amended or rejected because the Committee thinks that subjects' clinical welfare is not otherwise properly protected, and if this happens then the public may reasonably wish to know that it happens. Such information would indicate the committee's competence, vigilance and resolution. Furthermore, and within the limits set by reasonable commercial and scientific confidentiality, researchers and sponsors whose cooperation with the REC leads to the approval of amended protocols will enjoy public recognition of their responsible attitude towards clinical research. By the same token, and within the same constraints, there seems to be no good reason why the public should not know when a particular sponsor or researcher is unable to comply with the proper requirements of ethical review. Moreover it is clearly a matter of proper public interest that the occurence, if not all the clinical details, of difficulties in recruiting subjects, of subsequent adverse events or of the withdrawal of patients should be on record, as should the steps the REC has taken with regard to monitoring trial results and publications. To do this job properly requires a properly managed and properly maintained database (something which contributes more generally to good practice in ethical review).

Finally, it is in the interests of a continuing and evolving understanding of research ethics and of ethical review, that the public should be able to grasp and assess for themselves the sorts of considerations which their REC thinks important. The educative rôle of RECs, about which more will be said in Section 8.5, is one which can be promoted through the publication of an Annual Report – but only if the Report contains sufficient detail as to be meaningful.

7.6   Commercial confidentiality and the public interest

> *It is because we put up with bad things that*
> *hotel-keepers continue to give them to us.*
> (Anthony Trollope)

It's worth reminding ourselves that a conflict between commercial and public interests is one of the reasons why we need ethical review in the first place, so we shouldn't be dismayed by being confronted with this conflict anew. Much commercial interest is clearly legitimate, and if there is no substantial reason to the contrary, then commercial confidentiality should be respected. Most new medicines are developed in a competitive commercial environment, and without commercial confidentiality (at least under present conditions), much of the relevant commercial activity would simply not take place and to that extent clinical medicine and patient care would be the poorer. On the other hand, no consideration is ever proof against absolutely all others, and we can imagine situations where the public interest should prevail over the interests of commercial confidentiality. The question is whether such a situation need ever arise in the course of ethical review of clinical research. What this amounts to is whether the mechanisms of clinical research ever require the breaking of commercial confidentiality. Such situations would arise only rarely, such as where there arose an overwhelming need for further *ad hoc* scientific peer review outside the particular commercial community concerned, for instance in response to newly emergent questions about the safety of an investigation that was already under way. Of course this requires us to form a judgement on the proper extent and scope of public accountability of the REC. Does proper accountability require that proceedings and associated minutes should be public property? If so, then this would mean jeopardising commercial confidentiality, as rival firms could scrutinise the minutes of, or even attend, REC meetings considering each others' frontline research, complete with scientific details[8]. However, without access to copies of the Committee's agenda and other preparatory papers or more particularly to actual protocols, the details contained in Committee minutes would in scientific and commercial terms be scanty; as a route to serious industrial espionage, records of the REC's deliberations appear unpromising. Nevertheless, if even the threat of such a hazard would seriously inhibit commercial involvement in research (and perhaps this needs to be demonstrated rather than simply assumed) then it would count significantly against making the meetings or detailed proceedings of RECs a public affair. But this is not the only consideration in that question.

Another, perhaps more serious, possibility is that if and when things went wrong in the conduct of a research project and if more particularly research subjects were harmed, then a further review process might need to take account of commercially sensitive details, and might conceivably need to do so in an open hearing. However, this is of course a possibility inherent in the present system, in that actions for damages are always a possibility and such sensitive details might conceivably be relevant there as well.

7.7   The public REC meeting?

All professions are conspiracies against the laity.
(George Bernard Shaw)

At first sight the considerations here involve, roughly, the tension between on the one hand the legitimate public interest in monitoring a process that is carried out in the public name and for the protection of the public good, and on the other hand the legitimate private interests in defending commercial and scientific advantage in the pursuit of success – a success which, after all, is the main driving force behind the production of many beneficial substances and techniques used in clinical care. If adequate monitoring of the process can be carried out without jeopardising the relevant private interests, then it would be wrong to insist, for no good reason, on inhibiting these putative advances in patient care by imposing unnecessary constraints. The question then reverts to whether in fact adequate monitoring can be done without public access to meetings and minutes, and we shall return to this presently.

Beyond these considerations, however, the Department of Health's *Guidelines* draw attention to another possible reason for maintaining the confidentiality of meetings and minutes. This concerns the freedom of discussion available to the members of the REC. We may take it as self-evidently true that members will be more free to discuss a research proposal frankly if they are not required to do so in the presence of the researcher or proposer. By the same token, and applying it considerably more extensively, the *Guidelines* take the view that free and frank discussion requires a more general privacy, and that the meetings should therefore be private and the minutes confidential to the Committee[9]. The need for uninhibited discussion does provide a strong reason for respecting the privacy of meetings and minutes, since the REC members should feel perfectly able to resist pressure, real or imagined, to approve research against the interests of the research subjects. This means that on both sides of this question of public REC hearings there is now an argument which is couched essentially in terms of protecting the research subject. However we ought to remember that the present argument about privacy cuts both ways. A private discussion need not be one which by its very nature favours the interests of the research subjects; on the contrary the presently higher profile, of properly constituted RECs and of ethical review as a subject of public interest and debate, in part reflects the fact that in the past private discussions have been too vulnerable to promoting the wrong interests.

However, this objection can be perhaps be met: what was wrong in the past was not necessarily that the discussions of ethics committees were held in private, but that they were not always being conducted by the most appropriate people. The privacy of discussion might be said to accentuate the direction the discussion would tend to take anyway; too cosy a group of senior clinical researchers may have their ethical instincts subdued by privacy, just as by the same token too sceptical or – as one might put it – too 'bolshy' a group of laymen might similarly be given too much room for sheer icon-bashing by the luxury of discussions in camera, with no public scrutiny beyond a mere list of judgements. (As against this, being provided with an audience can similarly bring out the worst in the iconoclast.) The point is that, if conducted by the appropriate people, the discussion should not be led astray simply by being conducted in private.

To summarise, then, it seems that public confidence in good ethical review consists first in confidence that it is being carried out by the appropriate people, and second in having just sufficient access to the details of the procedures as to appreciate the general competence and seriousness with which the discussion is conducted – without in the process needlessly inhibiting either the frankness and sincerity of the discussion or the commercial confidence in which research is placed before the Committee. It is therefore likely that, provided sufficient information concerning the two matters just listed, namely appropriate membership and competent and serious discussion, is put before the public in some form (probably a significantly more substantial Annual Report), the advantages of public access to meetings and minutes are outweighed by the disadvantages.

Notes

1   Department of Health, *Local Research Ethics Committees*, London: Department of Health (1991), para. 2.10.

2   *ibid.*, para. 2.7.

3   This is a reasonable inference from the socio-geographic distribution of disease, disability and injury. For an indictment of the situation to be found in the United Kingdom, see Black, D., *Inequalities in Health*, Harmondsworth: Penguin (1982).

4   Department of Health, *op. cit.*, para. 1.1.

5   *ibid.*, para. 2.8.

6   *ibid.*, para. 2.4.

7   *ibid.*, para. 2.16.

8   Interestingly, the legislature in Denmark are pondering this very problem at the time of writing. A new law is being considered which would put the proceedings of ethics committees into the public domain, but its drafting is being qualified by the need to preserve commercial confidentiality: we are grateful to Dr Søren Holm for this information.

9   Department of Health, *op. cit.*, para. 2.15.

Chapter Eight

Good ethical review in practice

8.1   Criteria for good practice

He could never quite make up his mind about a new
symphony until he had seen the composer's mistress.
(H.L. Mencken)

The whole point of ethical review of clinical research is to ensure the safety and best interests of research subjects.   Whilst review committees should encourage the execution of good research and, arguably, stimulate and guide researchers in drawing up decent research proposals, neither of these aims should threaten or compromise the fundamental duty of such committees to protect research subjects.   As a result the review should be seen to be **independent**, **comprehensive** and **thorough**.

An analogy with the judicial processes of the lower courts in the United Kingdom may help us here.   In such courts magistrates, who are neither expected nor encouraged to have specialist legal qualifications, hear evidence from qualified attorneys, and receive guidance from a legally qualified clerk on points of law; having done so, they then determine the verdict upon the accused and, where necessary, pass sentence.   Here justice must not only be done but must also be seen to be done so that the public be reassured.   In order to achieve this kind of public confidence magistrates are not allowed to consider the cases of people who are known to them.   They might of course be capable of maintaining a judiciously impartial mind in such cases, but the public would not be assured of this.   So the judgements must always be seen to be independent of any mutual interests of the judges and the judged.   In addition the magistrates must be seen to have the opportunity to take into account all the issues at stake. Rules of evidence insist that judgements be based on the facts presented in court and on nothing else. In addition magistrates are entitled to ask of witnesses whatever questions will assist their understanding of points made by both prosecution and defence attorneys. Clearly it would not be in the interests of justice for verdicts to be based on the prejudices or whims of an uncomprehending bench of magistrates. Connectedly it is crucial for them to have enough time to consider matters in sufficient detail to reach sound verdicts. In the British legal system the term 'summary trial' is reserved for cases heard in the lower courts; but this is a technical term and is certainly not meant to imply a lack of thoroughness in the presentation and weighing of evidence.

It is true that ethical review is not a legal requirement in most countries and even where it is it does not take the form of a legal proceeding. Nevertheless there are useful lessons to be learned from the judicial analogy. The point of both processes is to protect the public, and the public needs to be assured that this is happening. In ethical review as in judicial hearings, serious judgements have to be made; whilst there are no experts in morality as such, nonetheless members of review committees have to adopt a judicious frame of mind and exercise precisely the kind of care demanded of members of the judicial bench.

8.2   The question of independence

Those who have free seats at the play hiss first.
(Chinese proverb)

We have already considered in section 7.2 the importance of proper representation in the membership of an ethical review committee. In ensuring that the committee membership can draw on a wide range of experience including the experience of professional groups it is nevertheless important to make sure that members keep their critical independence as individuals. Whilst the expert insights of the committee's various clinical specialists are valuable in connection with any given research project, these insights must be kept strictly apart from any mutual interests of researchers and reviewers.

Historically, hospital-based ethics committees in Britain involved consultants from different specialisms, considering each others' applications in short meetings with over-full agendas; too often the proposers and the scrutineers were simply the same people. With hindsight it was always likely that the earliest procedural scrutiny of proposed research would have been moulded by the assumptions prevalent within a hierarchical system of medical administration. Just as the scientific quality of proposed research was subjected to peer review within a well-defined structure of professional seniority, so the natural form of the earliest ethical review processes would have appeared to be a comparable peer review process. Within organised health care provision, the various relationships of mutual and one-way dependence which gave rise to what now appears a somewhat fragile approach to ethical review would also have inhibited both recognition of its shortcomings and self-criticism regarding its continuance. The complex personal and professional relationships, both collaborative and competitive, between different clinicians would be further complicated by considerations of their relative seniority, questions of prestige, the imperatives of their research reputations, and perhaps even by matters of remuneration and the relationships between researchers and sponsors. As with any profession which has a tendency to close ranks, it would be naturally difficult for an REC largely composed of senior clinicians who either were responsible for or were themselves active researchers to simulate the sort of detachment necessary for effective ethical review. Without acting improperly in any conscious or intentional sense, professional colleagues could find it hard to view each others' research proposals with the sort of detachment that effective ethical review unquestionably needs.

This kind of conflict of interests is self-evident. But the line between reviewers' insights and their interests can be blurred in a number of other and more subtle ways. First, the **professional interests** of both the researcher and one or more reviewers may coincide. For example, a nurse member or general practitioner member may wish to see nursing research or general practice research respectively enjoy a higher general profile. These are worthy desires but they don't belong in sound evaluation of particular nursing or general practice research protocols. The members are not on the review committee to promote such professional interests. To allow such an intrusion would not only frustrate the protection of research subjects, it would also, inevitably, fail to realise its secondary aim. The research profile of a profession is not going to be enhanced by the approval of second-rate research protocols – indeed the reverse will be the result.

Second, the working interests of researchers and reviewers may overlap or be complementary. We have discussed the obvious danger when personnel who work in the same establishment or for the same sponsor review each others' research protocols. The complementary danger arises if the researcher and the reviewer happen to be competing for funds from a common source, or if the researcher is likely to move ahead significantly on a project that overlaps or competes with the committee member's own research. The subtle pressure such common interests might produce on the reviewer would also compromise sound review. In either of these sorts of cases there is a conflict of interests for the committee member; the UK Department of Health's *Guidelines* urge that:

> Any member of the LREC who has an interest which may affect
> their consideration of a particular research proposal should be

asked to declare that interest, and if necessary should temporarily
withdraw from the committee[1].

Third, the **management interests** of reviewers must not intrude upon the ethical
review of research protocols. In the United Kingdom the Department of Health
Guidelines explicitly rule out the Local Research Ethics Committees as a
management arm of the Health Authority to which they are accountable.   Whilst
ethical approval of a research protocol is a necessary qualification *en route* to
carrying out that research, the question of whether regional or local health budgets
can afford to pay for the research is a separate question which must be answered
by management authorities and not by the Research Ethics Committee.   So,
although it may be the responsibility of a funding authority to set up an ethical
review committee, the independence of that committee from management decisions
is crucial.   The constitutions of these committees should guarantee this
independence and the committees should insist on their independence being
respected by the commissioning Authority. Failure to do this will almost inevitably
mean either that some good research will be ruled out for improper reasons or, still
more serious, that some low quality research which promises management benefits
will be approved, perhaps against the research subjects' interests.   In this
connection we were especially troubled when it was reported to us recently that the
Chairmanship of a Local Research Ethics Committee had been imposed upon that
committee by the commissioning District Health Authority against the provisions
of the constitution of that committee, in order for the Authority to 'keep control of
the committee'.

8.3   The question of comprehensiveness

What after all is a halo? It's only one more thing to keep clean.
(Christopher Fry)

It is not easy to determine how much information should be produced to a
research ethics committee in order to guarantee that it is in possession of all the
information necessary to make a proper evaluation of a research protocol.   For
example, in Phase II trials the sponsoring company will provide a investigator's
brochure which contains all the papers relating to previous animal tests which
have been executed.   It will also contain all the details of storage of the
pharmaceutical substance to be tested and a host of details about record-keeping
and reporting.   None of this information can ever be entirely ruled out as
irrelevant to a proper review of the protocol. Some observations and questions

may arise in the committee's discussion, for example about the production of specific enzyme levels that could affect the research subjects' well-being, which could be illuminated by reference to the studies carried out on animals. At the very least a copy of the full investigator's brochure should be available at the review meeting for reference in such circumstances; the pharmacist member will typically be best placed to consult and interpret the brochure. This documentation should also be available for other phases of the development of pharmaceutical substances. However, it would be a waste of valuable time for all members of a committee to read all such papers for all trials. Indeed, it would be impossible. It is a great help to committees if a responsible summary of such work is available which details features about the tolerated dosages, toxicity and observed side effects of the use of the substance in this preliminary work. Summaries of this kind could be so valuable to a Committee that there is a good argument for moving towards the routine production of them as a part of a standard protocol[2]. Many pharmaceutical protocols do already include more general introductions or summaries from which a lot of this information can be extracted; it would not involve much extra work on the part of those sponsors and applicants who already take a responsible approach to the writing of protocols for them to provide a self-contained summary specifically for the ethical review process. As we shall see when we come to consider the *pro-forma* application form in Chapter Nine and multi-location research in Chapter Twelve, the efficiency benefits of putting key information in a standardised and readily-accessed form are relevant to the proposers of research as well as to its reviewers.

The presence of the researcher for interview is an invaluable aid in ensuring comprehensivenesss of review. His or her presence gives the committee an opportunity to press questions behind the information contained in the presented protocol. In addition, of course, it gives the committee an opportunity to assess the grasp which the researcher has of the trial in question – an important consideration which we shall pursue in more detail in considering multi-location research in Chapter Twelve. There will be occasions when the local researcher will not be in a position to answer some of the questions which the committee may wish to ask. When this happens the Committee must make sure that matters are not left open, but that written enquiries be made to the sponsoring company to clarify the issue and satisfy the committee. If there are numerous or particularly worrying questions to be asked, the committee should be free to request that a spokesperson for the sponsoring organisation appear at a subsequent meeting to satisfy the committee on the points at issue.

Alternatively there may be features of a trial which the researcher and sponsoring company feel perfectly happy about but which leave anxieties in the mind of the committee. The committee will be reluctant either to approve or to reject a protocol if the members lack the necessary knowledge to make a responsible judgement. In such cases comprehensive review depends on the possibility of the committee seeking the advice of an independent expert, as we pointed out in section 7.1, with the permission of the sponsor, before proceeding with the process of approval. Refusal by the sponsoring company to agree to such a request would be sufficient reason for the committee to refuse approval, preferring to err on the side of caution in order to protect the interests of the research subjects.

Like 'fully informed consent' the notion of fully comprehensive information is an illusion. In any research trial there will always be important unknowns and there will often be disagreement about which features, if any, constitute crucial objections to the acceptability of a protocol. The standard that has to be adopted must be parallel to the 'reasonable patient' standard in consent procedures. In other words, sufficient information for a reasonable judgement to be made must be provided by the researcher. Refusal by a researcher or sponsor to provide additional information requested by a committee will always count as a conclusive reason for that committee to refuse to approve a protocol.

Some documents will be absolutely essential to a decent research proposal. These will include a proper *pro-forma* application (see Chapter Nine), all relevant approval certificates such as a Clinical Trials Certificate or Clinical Trials Exemption, and of course a user-friendly information sheet for the research subject and a properly constructed consent form which will include, for example, full details of whether the proposed research carries indemnity (see section 10.3 below). In studies involving the use of questionnaires, a copy of the questionnaire should always be produced together with a copy of the letter of approach to the research subjects if they are to be contacted by post. (In the case of semi-structured interviews, precise documentation may not be possible; here the REC relies on direct questioning of the proposed researcher to make sure that intrusive and distressing lines of enquiry are not envisaged.) Another essential document is of course the memorandum of any financial agreement between the researcher and the sponsor, where one exists. Details should always be provided of payments for the research to both researchers and their respective research funds and departments, as should payments to research subjects. Details of all payments-in-kind should also be provided – for example, the provision of valuable pieces of equipment for use in the trial which afterwards will be donated, or leased or sold at very low cost, to the researchers or the units where the research is to be carried out. Similar considerations apply to administrative equipment such as computers, and also to research conference expenses and so on.

It is disappointing that the otherwise admirable recommendations of the European Forum for Good Clinical Practice (EFGCP)[3] should recommend in their section on required documentation for ethical review that ethics committees '…not require full disclosure of payments to investigators…'. This goes quite against their earlier recommendation that 'In cases where there is a potential conflict of interest, applicants are to disclose the nature of the potential conflict and describe the steps taken to minimise a bias [*sic*] reporting of results.' Clearly the level of remuneration paid to the investigator and the basis on which it is made can lead to obvious conflicts of interest. The REC can decide how to protect the interests of research subjects only when it is in full possession of such details.

8.4   The question of thoroughness

> *The opera ain't over till the fat lady sings.*
> (Dan Cook)

Ethical review of clinical research is worth nothing if it is not thorough. It will not do simply to guarantee the independence of all the reviewers and the comprehensiveness of the information provided if the process of review itself is less than thorough. Given the quite marked increase in the number of protocols reviewed by some Research Ethics Committees in the United Kingdom over the past two years, partly due to the amalgamation of various District Health Authorities, it has been reported that above five hundred protocols are reviewed by some single committees in a twelve-month period in monthly meetings[4]. An average of almost fifty protocols per meeting is, we think, ludicrous. However well qualified the committee may be, however well informed and however well serviced and chaired, it seems to us impossible that anything approaching an acceptable standard of review could be maintained with such workloads.

In our 1992 survey of British RECs we uncovered numerous unsatisfactory methods of review adopted by the newly constituted Local Research Ethics Committees as set out in the revised Department of Health *Guidelines*. These methods had evidently been adopted, by and large, to cope with having to process too large a number of protocols by the committees. (As the workloads have since then increased as described above it seems fair to suppose that there is even greater cause for concern now than at the time of our survey.) From among those that we came across, five of these questionable 'labour-saving devices' are presented below. We believe they constitute a potentially serious threat to the welfare of research subjects in the United Kingdom wherever they allow the appearance of proper subject protection to be maintained for public reassurance, because processes of which they are habitually a part cannot deliver that protection. Research subjects are placed in a more vulnerable position where there is merely the **appearance** of ethical review of clinical research than where there is none at all.

First, while **chairman's action** is a necessary possibility in certain circumstances, it should be available only to expedite decisions already made by the committee, or to resolve urgent matters shortly to be confirmed by the committee. An example of the former would occur when the Committee asks the chairman to authorise the progress of a trial that has been conditionally approved, once the relevant conditions – study modifications, the provision of further information or other provisos – have been met. The chairman would then be expected to report the supply of those additional features when reporting his action at the subsequent meeting of the committee. An example of the latter could occur when there is an amendment to a protocol for a trial already in progress; if delaying approval until the next meeting of the committee would seriously hinder the research or, alternatively, leave the subjects open to greater than minimal risk, then there is a clear case for chairman's action. However, it is crucial that any such action be reported to the committee for confirmation at the earliest opportunity. In the case of serious changes or the reporting of serious adverse events presenting a *prima facie* case for the suspension of a study, the chairman may wish to call an emergency meeting of the committee rather than take individual action. He or she may alternatively canvass the views of a number of members before taking chairman's action. Providing that they are brought to the next meeting of the Committee for confirmation, then such procedures don't amount to bypassing the Committee's due processes.

Not all chairman's action is taken with such care, however. We discovered one committee which met only a couple of times a year, largely for social purposes, and which conducted its business by telephone. The chairman simply obtained the 'all clear' from a number of members confirming his view that a given protocol was satisfactory. He assured us that he had 'no trouble' with his members. Such a procedure is obviously open to abuse and certainly rules out the possibility of thorough review in the form of detailed face-to-face discussion after careful scrutiny of papers. It is face-to-face discussion which so often throws up matters of concern that many members will not have noticed, or which enables the Committee to see how a combination of matters themselves not individually very significant can combine to form a worrying pattern. Without the context of a frank and open discussion such possibilities are diminished if not ruled out.

The above example was presented to us by its Chairman as a model committee; a similar picture was painted in the case of another Committee where meetings regularly occurred but always simply to confirm, or otherwise, the chairman's actions taken since the previous meeting. Whilst this is some improvement on the first variant of chairman's action, it still seems quite unsatisfactory for a number of reasons. Most obviously, if the Committee decided to reverse the Chairman's approval – clearly a possibility under this scheme – it might do so only to find that the research had already begun. If the problems lay with the approaches to potential subjects, selection of subjects, randomisation to placebo arms of trials and so on, then harm could be done to patients before the committee's veto becomes effective.

In each of the above cases chairman's action was taken without the benefit of an interview with the researcher before the full Committee, or of full discussion with the other Committee members. (The general case for establishing a committee as such is incompatible with the practice of relying on an inner circle of the chairman's *confidantes*.) If the committee happens to disagree with the chairman on some cases where it feels approval has been improperly given and on which it would wish to consult with the researcher, then a further problem presents itself. The researcher will need notice to attend the Committee, unless all researchers are required to turn up in what will often be a perfunctory manner – something researchers are unlikely to tolerate. Arranging the subsequent interview at proper notice will produce further delay and give rise to the dilemma of whether to suspend the trial in the interim period, producing a variety of problems including the need in some cases to recruit a new set of subjects, or to let it run even longer without proper approval. Neither alternative is acceptable and practices which give rise to such a dilemma must be discouraged.

Second, the holding of **inquorate meetings** is, like Chairman's action, a way of bypassing the Committee; procedures which are designed to do this are amongst the most serious threats to thorough review. Some members of committees who responded to our questionnaires concerning the need for training of members of British RECs indicated that they did not know whether their committee had a quorum provision in its constitution and even if it did they were ignorant of its nature. The minimum numbers and identities of members constituting a quorum are important to guarantee responsible consideration of a clinical research protocol.

Third, the provision of **inadequate information** to the committee will also prevent thorough review. The key component to any member's being properly prepared for the REC's meeting is that he or she should have had sufficient time to study properly the agenda papers, specifically the research protocols and their accompanying correspondence. Research protocols are often lengthy, complicated and demanding documents; furthermore they are by no means uniform (as the modes and areas of research are themselves not uniform) and, whilst members will gain experience in finding their way around certain more standardised kinds of protocol (for instance, many kinds of multi-centre drug trials), each fresh protocol requires careful attention to detail – some of it occasionally obscure even to medically qualified members – in order that the potential ethical pitfalls be identified and scrutinised. Important weaknesses, where there are any, are often to be found only in the fine detail of the proposal – for example in the amount of blood that is to be collected from a subject in the course of a trial, the number of X-rays to be taken, or in a combination of the exclusion criteria and the possible adverse events. Understanding research protocols requires time and concentration;

furthermore, being alert to possibly novel sources of ethical concern demands imagination from those reviewing the protocols themselves. The proper review of a protocol is not a five-minute matter, and with many committees considering upwards of fifteen or more protocols in a meeting, the agenda papers absolutely must be in the hands of Committee members well in advance of the meeting itself, in order that they have the proper opportunity to study them.

Similarly, the incompleteness of papers should not be treated lightly. Often the absence of a written consent form or a readable information sheet are accompanied by a promise to provide such documents to subjects at the recruitment stage. Clearly the committee should always insist on seeing such documents before final approval is given to proceed as they may be the source of serious objections to the trial. But beyond this there is a case for insisting that only properly documented applications should be considered at all, other than in quite exceptional circumstances. Revisiting applications to 'tie up the loose ends' at later meetings means that members must inevitably consider much of the substance of those applications more than once, and this is a sheer waste of everyone's time. Committees should not be afraid to stipulate their requirements to applicants; there is far more cause for researchers to feel disgruntled at delays caused by inefficient review procedures than there is at delays caused by their own failure to present properly documented submissions at the first time of asking.

There is obviously a compromise to be struck between the requirements of early circulation of the papers and the need to keep the Committee's deliberations up to date and topical – there is no virtue in first considering protocols six months after they have been submitted. However, it is reasonable for the Committee to specify an advance date by which protocols must have been received by the Committee's secretary in order for them to be considered at the next meeting. As a rough suggestion, our experience indicates that a full agenda requires papers to be received by members – not simply put in the mail – at least a clear week before meeting. This means, in practice, that the secretary should receive properly prepared submissions and their accompanying protocols, in full, at least a week before that in order to allow for duplication and distribution.

Proposals received subsequently should not automatically be tabled for consideration at the meeting in question, unless there is good reason to think that they can be properly considered. Tabling papers for consideration at some subsequent meeting is tantamount to deferring them anyway (with the possible advantage that members have them in their possession for a longer period; however whether in practice this means that they will receive better consideration than they would have received, when being examined in time set aside for the consideration of the agenda papers as a whole, is questionable).

Fourth, **unsatisfactory meetings** can also frustrate the thoroughness of ethical review. It is important to point out in the context of the question of thoroughness that the form of the meeting can hinder proper review. Over-full agendas are the main threat. Serious attention may be paid to protocols appearing early on the agenda and large numbers of later protocols may be nodded through by a weary Committee whose attention levels are declining. Those who are seasoned participants in different kinds of meetings and committees may recognise here a useful ploy enabling items which are important to the chair to slip through almost unnoticed at the end of meetings; whether or not this is ever really acceptable in any other contexts, it will certainly not do in ethical review of research. Of course the question now arises as to how many protocols are acceptable in a single REC meeting. The answer will depend on a number of variables, including of course the length and complexity of the protocols themselves but also on the timing of the meeting and its duration. For example, numbers of review meetings have been brought to our attention which are convened at lunchtimes, with the unhappy consequence of clinical members having to withdraw, to attend to their lists and clinics, before the decisions to approve the presented protocols are taken. Clearly if approval is given on such a basis then too many protocols have been included on the agenda. It is our experience and the experience of numerous members and chairpersons whom we have interviewed that any number above six typical-length protocols per hour imposes too great a strain on a Committee and provokes the temptation to consider protocols in a perfunctory fashion. Many meetings are convened to last between two and two-and-a-half hours. One such meeting per month would make possible a realistic maximum of about one hundred and seventy protocols per annum for a hard-working committee to consider properly. We think that any further demands should be met by duplicating review committees[5]; otherwise the activity of ethical review will fall into disrepute.

8.5   The importance of feedback

On an occasion of this kind it becomes more than a moral
duty to speak one's mind. It becomes a pleasure.
(Oscar Wilde)

In discussing the Committee's working procedures, the Department of Health *Guidelines* observe that 'when research proposals are rejected by the LREC, the reasons for that decision should be made available to the applicant'[6]. Of course, courtesy demands no less; however, we can give other good grounds for the importance of proper feedback. The REC tends to deal mainly with a restricted number of known local researchers, many of whom become familiar to the Committee through repeated submissions of different research projects. It is obviously in the interests of potential research subjects and of the REC itself, no less than in those of the researcher, that the researcher should have every opportunity to appreciate and share the moral values that are at stake in the processes of ethical review and in the decisions that the REC takes.

Furthermore there is no reason why this should be confined simply to advice accompanying requests for amendment, much less just to outright rejections. Research which is approved but which comes from a researcher not well known to the REC offers an opportunity for the Committee to express specific approval or appreciation of the way in which the ethical challenges of the research have been met in its design. In this way the REC can help the researcher to establish or to consolidate good ethical practices which will serve everyone's interests well in the course of future research proposals. Although feedback takes time, it will in all likelihood save more future time than it presently consumes; protocols which are approved outright take considerably less of the REC's time than protocols which have to make a second or even third appearance with amendments, or whose approval has to be made conditional on some revision or on the supply of further information. If only from a sense of enlightened self-interest, the REC has a stake in researchers 'getting it right first time', as often as this can be done. But of course the researcher herself has an interest in precisely this, and should feel entitled to expect that the REC will help her in this regard.

There is a general point arising from these considerations. The researcher has certain reasonable expectations regarding the way she is dealt with by her REC, and these expectations are the more reasonable when we consider that they ultimately bear on the way that research subjects are routinely regarded, and on the efficiency with which the research process can be translated into better patient care. But if this is true, then patients, the research subject population and indeed the general public can reasonably share the expectation that the REC will not merely select but **promote** ethically sound research. In short, the REC itself has a rôle in the continuing education of the research community with regard to good ethical design of clinical research.

There may indeed be a case for formalising this rôle at some stage, and for inviting newer researchers (or recalcitrant ones!) to meet the REC and its members, to take part in discussion and debate about ethical issues away from the naturally difficult context of trying to get approval for their own individual research projects. Once again the point is worth making that investment of the REC's energies here may well lead to more appropriate research submissions in the future, which in turn leads to a more efficient use of the REC's time and to a quicker response for the researcher – with all that that implies in terms of expediting the research itself.

8.6   The REC's sanctions

If you don't like my story get out of the punt.
(James Joyce)

What happens when research is not ethically satisfactory?   The REC's difficulties here lie in the fact that the character of a proposed research is not fixed once-and-for-all.   The practical execution of what is on paper an exemplary proposal may turn out to be unacceptable, and ethical review requires us to be able to discover when this happens and to do something about it.   Not only are the interests of the current subjects of research threatened by the lack of surveillance but potential recruits for further trials are also put at risk when those trials are to be undertaken by researchers who fail to comply with approved protocols or to report adverse events, withdrawals and incomplete or aborted trials.

Within its terms of reference (in Britain, these refer to research which involves National Health Service patients, staff or facilities) even the merely advisory REC effectively has the power to prevent research which it considers inappropriate from being started;   its advice to the executive authorities in question is unlikely to be ignored.   When by contrast the REC's advice is that a particular research project meets acceptable ethical standards, we should be clear that this endorses only the intentions and commitments of the proposer of the research at the time of application.   Initial ethical approval is not a guarantee that all will be well, and hence the responsibilities of good ethical review do not end with the Committee's initial verdict.   The British Department of Health *Guidelines* clearly envisage a limited monitoring role for the REC, as an integral part of its functioning, in order to ensure that the ethical safeguards and undertakings in a proposal, and on which the ethical approval is grounded, are in fact carried out in practice[7].   If this important rôle properly falls to the local REC then it has enormous implications for the resourcing of Committees.   For the moment it's salutory to note that in our 1992 survey, 69% of the individual REC members who responded mistakenly believed that monitoring formed no part of the REC's rôle. The realities of current resourcing do nothing to correct this misperception.

On the presently rather large assumption that the monitoring functions can meaningfully be discharged in some way, the next question obviously concerns the enforcement of standards.   Presently the sanctions open to a British REC are these: withdrawal of ethical approval, and notification of the Health Authority that this has been done – this should lead, as a management decision by the Health Authority, to the trial being stopped forthwith, of which more below;   on occasion, reporting the researcher by name to his/her respective professional body notifying that body of the withdrawal of ethical approval and the breach on which that withdrawal is based; and on occasion, notification of the withdrawal to the publishers of any results arising from that research. However, these sanctions apply only to research which is conducted within the auspices of Health Authority personnel and facilities as presently envisaged by the Department of Health *Guidelines*, and obviously cannot apply to – and hence cannot protect the subjects of – research carried out outside those auspices. The responsibility for acting on the REC's advice and subsequent reports lies of course with the employer and with the professional body concerned. It is not clear whether any more direct sanctions on the part of the REC are desirable; however the REC certainly has a responsibility to exercise the sanctions which it does have, in the appropriate circumstances. When serious adverse events occur, and are not acted upon by the researcher or are not recognised as having general implications, it is possible that research which should be stopped forthwith in fact continues by default.

Mechanisms are obviously needed to make sure that research which ought to be stopped is in fact stopped. The British REC has no direct powers at present to do this, even when the information on which such a decision might be based is available. However, in withdrawing ethical approval it is open to the REC as an advisory body to advise and request that the Health Authority intervene to stop the trial in the clinical interests of the research subjects, if it is suspected that there is a need to do so. The problem at present is that it is not clear how those circumstances can ordinarily be identified, except by the pure chance of casual or coincidental, and inevitably private, report of untoward circumstances, made by a third party to a member of the REC. In effect, then, responsibility for stopping research when it is necessary or appropriate to do so rests virtually entirely with the researcher himself. Whilst this responsibility might no doubt be exercised perfectly properly by the overwhelming majority of researchers, it is not these but the small minority of irresponsible researchers with which the REC should be most concerned in this connection, since it is these researchers' subjects who are most in need of protection. This is a completely unsatisfactory basis for the monitoring of research: frankly, unless and until this problem is overcome, those who are probably the most vulnerable research subjects lack protection to that extent.

8.7   The problem of resources

She was a singer who had to take any note
above A with her eyebrows.
(Montague Glass)

This brings us inevitably to the question of resourcing. The proper monitoring and follow-up and policing of research is a necessary job to be done by somebody, but it is not clear that physical inspections can – or even ought to –

be done by a voluntary, non-executive, advisory body like the REC. Robust mechanisms of monitoring are needed, but perhaps these should be reporting directly (and swiftly) to the Chair of the REC. The same considerations of subject protection which make it inappropriate for Chairmen to give executive approval of a protocol suggest by contrast that it would be perfectly appropriate for Chairmen to take rapid executive action to halt or suspend improper research. The need to stop inappropriate research quickly is rarely mirrored by a convincing need to get research started abruptly. In section 11.4 we will look in more detail at the mechanisms of monitoring which are available to RECs at the moment.

Beyond the question of follow up, there are other substantial resource issues: secretarial support for the existing activities of RECs is probably provided through the Health Authority by simple diversion of existing administrative facilities, whose costs are buried in someone else's budget. But this demeans and undervalues the process of ethical review, as well as subjecting it to arbitrary and probably invisible cost restraints. The servicing of REC members needs to be as prompt and efficient as that of any other body contributing to patient welfare, which the REC is surely intended to. The advance circulation of agenda papers is often the first thing to be compromised by administrative resource limitations, yet we have already recognised that late circulation of papers itself severely compromises members' preparation for the REC meeting proper. The proper recruitment, induction and training of new committee members, together with continuing in-service training for existing members, can scarcely be even considered if the paperwork exhausts the committee's resources. And we have not yet considered the question of the merely honorary status of REC chairpersons and members. All the services of members of local RECs and central ethical review committees have, until recently, been voluntary. The honorary status of membership of these committees is now being called into question. Some chairpersons of review committees have recently begun to be paid for their services; surprisingly, the Department of Health *Guidelines* are silent on this important issue. The question of payments to ordinary committee members is also now becoming a pressing issue as Hospital Trusts and General Practices, for example, often resent the fact that their clinical employees must devote as much as one whole working day per month to examining research protocols and discussing them in Committee deliberations. As a result it is becoming increasingly difficult to make the best appointments to such local RECs. We suspect that this pressure will grow, but under the current resourcing constraints it is bound to exacerbate all the other resourcing problems of the REC. In short, it is hard for ethical review to be undertaken seriously – indeed, even **taken** seriously by those whom it affects – under these circumstances.

Ultimately the solution must simply be that new money be found. We shall briefly consider in section 12.4 below one possible funding solution involving a levy on research sponsors for the review of their protocols. The problems of such a solution, as we'll see, chiefly devolve onto the need for a central apparatus for administering it; but if ethical review is to be taken more seriously it will require commitment at the level of the national administration of health care provision.

8.8   The provision of training for reviewers

When I find myself in the company of scientists, I feel like a shabby curate
who has strayed by mistake into a drawing-room full of dukes.
(W.H. Auden)

In our 1992 survey of the members of RECs we established that there was a widespread feeling among members that they were insufficiently equipped for the job they were asked to do[8]. For instance, a significant majority of individual respondents said that they found it either very difficult or fairly difficult to assess scientific protocols (73.6% of respondents), to assess trial designs (64.9%) and to identify the risks and benefits of a particular proposal (70.5%). We asked them about the importance of providing specific training in specific areas of their work, and clear majorities thought that such training was either very important or fairly important in terms of an introduction to ethical analysis (94.7%), a guide to trial design (84.5%), problem areas of ethical review (97.1%) and even the proper terms of reference of ethical review (76.9%). There was a striking degree of agreement betwen the professional clinicians and the other members, including the lay members, in terms of their view of their own needs and abilities.   Effective ethical review is a demanding business, making heavy requirements of individual members in terms of time, concentration, discretion, knowledge, experience and sensitive and often imaginative judgement, and requiring them also to bring these qualities together and to function as a team in REC discussions and decisions.   In terms of the relevant clinical knowledge, the clinical members of the REC start at an obvious advantage over the lay members, who have to gather much of the required understanding as they go along; but clearly even the clinical members need not **as individuals** have all the relevant knowledge from different clinical areas, and they too must learn the skill of identifying and obtaining from other sources items or areas of knowledge which they do not themselves possess.

However, there is a further area in which all Committee members start on a more or less equal footing, and that is the area of expertise in ethical understanding and judgement in relation to clinical research. As Jonathan Miller puts it, 'We are all PhDs in morals'; no-one has an advantage in moral judgement simply in virtue of his or her professional training. Nevertheless, skills beyond those of the conduct and negotiations of ordinary daily life are needed in the special moral context of clinical research, and these are concerned with understanding the morally relevant features of different kinds of research, research which gives rise to characteristic moral challenges regarding the protection of the research subject's interests. This is a matter not simply of knowing where these features might be, but of appreciating what they can mean for the research subject. In this regard, once the lay member has a broad grasp of the different kinds of research, then she is equally well placed with her clinical colleagues to grapple with the seriousness of the moral challenge which the research represents, and of course to pick out and to weigh similar features in subsequent research proposals.

To illustrate the point, consider what we said about the weighing of risks and benefits in Chapter Five. Some of the risks will be more readily spotted by the professional clinician, though often even she will have to resort to more specialised advice. However, once the risks have been identified, the question of what they mean in human terms, and how (if at all) they can be traded against the benefits, is not in itself a medical matter at all. This is a complicated, elusive and evaluative matter, and it requires both imagination and experience – something that will be gained as readily by the lay member as by the clinical member.

Ethical review in practice requires in the REC member the development both of knowledge and of the kind of judgement that is honed by experience. The newly appointed member is thrust into a responsible rôle, typically without the slightest formal preparation. Our survey showed, however, that even established clinical members of committees feel that they lack various kinds of expertise and confidence in coming to decisions. (Moreover many felt that they lacked – even after a period of service on a committee – the abilities needed to make their contributions felt in discussion. And not all chairmen regarded themselves as well equipped to perform their especially difficult and sensitive rôles.)

The process of gaining experience can be facilitated, accelerated and potentiated by the provision of suitable training at the right time. We noted some areas in respect of which respondents to our survey expressed the need for training. In addition to these, substantial proportions saw a need for training in the matter of the conduct of Committee meetings (53.1%), the proper constitution of RECs (45.8%) and the development of members' own communication skills in discussion (43.4%). (Our subsequent Report to the Department of Health included suggested training materials which could be used to address precisely these needs[8].) There seems no doubt that the effectiveness of ethical review depends on the effectiveness of REC members, individually and collectively, and that some formal preparation can significantly improve the effectiveness of both newly appointed and established REC members.

There are various ways in which that training could be provided, and we can mention two ways in which we have had substantial involvement: (i) the large-scale residential training conference at which members from RECs all over the country gather for an intensive programme of lectures and workshops; and (ii) the running of a series of linked workshops for the members of a single REC, on separate days over a specified period. Each has its advantages and disadvantages, of course. Also, there is some difference between training aimed at the initial preparation of newly-appointed members, and training aimed at supplementing or 'refreshing' the skills and expertise of established members. Again, the rôle of chairman carries specific requirements and responsibilities, and a good case can be made for both in-service training for existing chairmen and preparatory training for those who are likely future chairmen. The nature of the training event must obviously reflect its aims. Both the large-scale conference and the workshop sequence which we have described can be 'loaded' towards the needs of either established or newly-appointed members; indeed, where these needs overlap – and they often do – then there are some advantages in combining both new and established members in the same training process, provided this is done with careful attention to those respects in which their needs also differ. (New members, both clinicians and lay-people, appreciate instruction on the varieties of research methodology, for instance.)

Other training methods exist, but not all are successful. American Institutional Review Board members have in many cases been provided with a series of excellently devised and impressively produced instructional videos, yet the reported benefits from them are low – chiefly, it appears, because IRB members find it more difficult to set aside the time and energy to engage in their own training on an isolated, individual basis. Just as ethical discussion is necessarily a collective matter, we suspect that effective training in ethical review requires the mutual encouragement and enthusiasm which is obtained only by collective training.

Virtually everyone agrees that proper formal training of REC members is necessary, but concerted means of funding this training are not forthcoming. In the United Kingdom, many District Health Authorities pay for individual REC members to attend large training conferences such as those we have described, and a few Health Authorities have funded workshop series dedicated to their own Committees. However, training costs money – like effective ethical review as such. And as we've seen, the means of providing this money have yet to be found. The **case** for providing it, however, remains.

Notes

1   *Guidelines*, para. 3.23.

2   Against this it might be objected that a summary written by the investigator could never be free of subjective bias. We are grateful to Dr. Peter Dewland for this observation.

3   European Forum for Good Clinical Practice (EFGCP), *Guidelines and Recommendations for European Ethics Committees*, Brussels: EFGCP, (June 1995), p. 7.

4   Alberti, K.G.M.M., 'Local research ethics committees: time to grab the bull by the horns', Editorial, *British Medical Journal*, 311 (1995), p. 640.

5   This principle has been adapted by one British REC with which we are familiar, which was constituted as a Joint Ethics Committee having overall responsibility for the working of a number of smaller panels, each of which considered a more manageable portion of the original workload.

6   Department of Health, *Local Research Ethics Committees*, London: Department of Health (1990), para. 2.12.

7   *ibid.*, para. 2.14.

8   Evans, D., (ed.) *Report on the Training Needs of Members of Local Research Ethics Committees*, Swansea: Centre for Philosophy and Health Care (1992).

Chapter Nine

The *pro-forma* application form and its requirements

9.1   General questions in plain language

*'Turbot, Sir', said the waiter, placing before me two
fishbones, two eyeballs and a bit of black macintosh.*
(Thomas Earle Welby)

Just as in the case of the patient information sheet for research subjects, where
we saw that it is possible to identify and to address the subject's reasonable
concerns in plain language, so too the REC's *pro-forma* application form can be
designed to obtain plain language answers to all the reasonable and foreseeable
concerns of the Committee.   The *pro-forma* provides a framework for
immediately identifying the ethically significant features of any research
protocol, enabling the REC to form a rapid overall appreciation of where their
discussion should be focused.   Of course, whereas a specific patient information
sheet is tailored to the details of a particular piece of proposed research, the *pro-
forma* has to be flexible enough to cover a wide range of different kinds of
research proposal, from retrospective studies of patient records to prospective
controlled clinical experiments.   But this variety can be accommodated quite
easily, by providing a comprehensive set of questions and then directing
applicants to respond to only those questions which are relevant to their
proposed research, and to identify and mark non-relevant questions as such.

The general concerns of the REC can be set out much as we set out the
general concerns of the prospective research subject.   There are of course rather
many of them, since they must anticipate the issues arising in many different

possible kinds of research proposal. The questions are dictated first and foremost by the concerns we have been discussing in Chapters Three, Five and Six. These concerns prompt at least the following questions, all of which ought ideally to be covered in a general-purpose *pro-forma*:

(a) Questions about the general aims and conduct of the research

- what is the proposed research project's title and/or reference number, for reliable future identification?

- what is the object of the research?

- who will be responsible for carrying out the research locally?

- who will be responsible for overseeing the central coordination of multi-location research?

- what premises and facilities will be used locally? Will their use involve resource implications for the local health authority?

- what other research will the applicant(s) be engaged in concurrently with the proposed research?

- will the research involve contact with patients or healthy volunteers? If so, how many?

- will the research involve subjects from any of the following groups: infants or children, foetuses, pregnant women, the frail elderly, the terminally ill, psychiatric patients, the mentally impaired? If so, would the research be impossible without using such patients?

- will the research involve access to confidential information about patients?

- will the research involve the administration of drugs, gases or vaccines?

- will the research involve the use of radioactive substances?

- will the research involve the use of invasive diagnostic or investigative procedures such as x-rays, biopsies or endoscopies?

- how long is the research intended to last?

- in prospective (experimental) research, what are the trial's end points? What criteria are there for stopping the trial early?

- what other similar or relevant research has been done in the past?

(b) Questions about the formal status of trial products

- if drugs, gases or vaccines are to be used, have they an associated clinical trial certificate (CTC) or clinial trial exemption certificate (CTX)? If so, what are the certificates' numbers and who can provide official confirmation of them?

- do any such products have a product licence?

- will they be used for approved indications? If so, what?

- will they be used for new indications? If so, what?

(c) Questions about the use of controls in prospective (experimental) research

- does the research involve the use of controls?

- if so, will subjects in the control group receive active treatment?

- if they will receive active treatment, is this treatment the recognised best existing or standard treatment? If not, why not, and how is the deviation justified?

- is the trial placebo controlled? If so, and if active comparator treatments are available, what justification is there for using placebo as comparator?

- if there are any subjects who will receive only placebo, are they at any clinical risk through being without active treatment during the relevant period of the trial?

- how will subjects be distributed between the primary study group(s) and the control group(s)? Is the distribution to be randomised?

- is there a washout period prior to the start of the trial? If there is, are subjects at any clinical risk through being without active treatment during the washout period?

- will the research be conducted on a single-blind, double-blind or open basis?

(d) Additional questions about the well-being of research subjects

- what discomforts, side effects or other harms might be expected by the research subjects?

- what precautions will be taken to minimise the effects of likely or possible harms arising in the course of the research?

- how will adverse events be identified? How will they be responded to?

- in the case of double-blinded research, what code-breaking provisions are there to deal with adverse events?

- are there any invasive diagnostic procedures which will be performed to meet the requirements of the research? If so, to what extent would these have been required in the ordinary clinical management of the patient outside the context of the proposed research?

- what provisions are made for compensating research subjects in the event of non-negligent harms arising from the research? What indemnity arrangements are in place for the researchers or their employing authority?

(e) Questions about the recruitment of subjects

- what is the envisaged age range of the research subjects?

- what in summary are the principal inclusion and exclusion criteria?

- is there a minimum number of subjects to be recruited locally before the research can begin?

- how will subjects be approached? Will they be recruited through hospital or GP patient lists?

- will they be approached through the clinician responsible for the aspect of their care which is relevant to the proposed research?

- will their GP be informed or consulted before the subjects are approached?

- will they be approached by letter? If so, is a copy of the letter included in the application to the REC?

- will subjects be offered any payment or other consideration in return for taking part? If so, what?

- will subjects be told that taking part in the research offers them any clinical benefits? If so, what?

(f) Questions about information and consent

- will the research involve any subjects who are likely to be unable to consent on their own behalf to taking part in the project (legally incompetent subjects)?

- if so, who is it envisaged will be required to give consent for them? In such cases, does the proposed research involve active treatment for **all** the participating subjects?

- where research involves legally incompetent subjects, is their participation necessary to the research?

- in the case of randomised trials, will patients clearly understand from these documents that their treatment will be determined randomly?

- in the case of placebo-controlled trials, will subjects clearly understand that they may not receive active treatment?

- is a copy of the proposed information sheet and consent form included in the application to the REC?

(g) Questions about financial implications

- will the investigator (or her clinical premises, facilities or specialism) receive financial payment for conducting the research?

- if so, is this made clear to participating subjects before they agree to take part?

- what is the total sum payable in the event of completing the study? To whom is it payable?

- where payment will be made to an endowment or trust fund for local research or education, who administers the fund?

- is there a minimum number of patients to be recruited before any remuneration can be made?

- will remuneration be made on a *per capita* basis, that is, payment for each patient recruited into and conducted through the research?

- are there any investigative, diagnostic or therapeutic procedures for which payment will be received on an itemised basis?

- is a copy of the financial agreement included in the application to the REC?

9.2 Saving time by taking pains

If at first you don't succeed, try, try again. Then quit.
No use bein' a damn fool about it.
(W.C. Fields)

A formal document setting out all of these questions individually, with adequate space for decent replies, would be rather long; but of course most applications would require responses to only a selection of the questions. In any case the completed document would be both much shorter and, from the REC member's perspective, far more pertinent and accessible than the average protocol. (Here we will leave open the matter of how the questions and their responses are physically set out, whether they will involve the ticking of boxes, physically typing out answers on the original *pro-forma* itself, word-processing files on diskette and so forth. This is largely a matter for the convenience and preference of the individual REC, although in section 12.2 we shall discuss the important advantages of a single uniform *pro-forma* application form for all RECs involved in the review of multi-location research.)

One extremely comprehensive version of a *pro-forma* application form is presented and discussed by Doyal who argues that despite its length it will save time for the applicant as well as the Committee, by preventing time-consuming delays caused by inadequate or incomplete initial applications[1]. In general we share his view, although a point will be reached at which an over-detailed *pro-forma* loses the advantages of a succinct focus for the benefit of REC members; it is arguable whether Doyal's version approaches this point. However, he is certainly right to think that researchers stand to benefit from getting their applications right first time. Moreover we think it is important that, in having to provide specific responses to the questions, the applicant to the REC is obliged to consider these dimensions of the research for herself. Time spent on this at the application stage is time well spent for the conscientious researcher, who should be considering these matters both before and during the conduct of the research itself. For this reason – let alone the risk of a wholly natural exasperation on the part of REC members – responses along the lines of 'See the accompanying protocol' should firmly be disallowed; RECs are entitled to insist on properly presented and properly supported applications, and should make it clear that applications which are not satisfactorily presented will not be considered.

Doyal[1] also makes the point, which we endorse, that requiring applicants to fill in a checklist of supporting documentation is an effective way of ensuring that their applications are properly complete on first submission. Again people will disagree over whether all the items on his list are essential to effective and efficient review. We think the following documentation is a minimum requirement:

- the full protocol;

- all letters of initial approach to subjects;

- copy of the letter to the subject's general practitioner (or Works Medical Officer if appropriate);

- all relevant information sheets (for patients/subjects, and/or their parents or guardians or other proxies);

- all relevant consent forms (as above);

- any financial agreements, including a statement of the administration of endowment or other funds for local use;

- all relevant CTCs/CTXs;

- a full specification of any compensation and indemnity provisions.

The important point about the *pro-forma* is that it offers a ready guide to identifying and appraising the key points of the proposed research – which is authoritatively specified in the supporting documents. Whilst the *pro-forma* carries the applicant's signature, its standing outside the REC's proceedings is merely informal. What counts, in legal and contractual terms, are first and foremost these other documents. That is why the *pro-forma* is no substitute for them. It is, however, an absolutely invaluable way of making those formal documents accessible and meaningful, if it is well designed and properly completed. As such it gives structure and backbone to the researcher's contruction of her proposal, to the Committee members' preparation, and to the REC's ethical discussion itself.

9.3 The case for standardisation

> *Opera in English is, in the main, just about*
> *as sensible as baseball in Italian.*
> (H.L. Mencken)

In this chapter we have been concerned with the general means to a uniformly high standard of applications to RECs. Here, this has been essentially a matter of substance rather than of style. In Chapter Twelve, when we come to consider the specific problems arising from research that is simultaneously carried out in several locations, we will see that there is also a strong case for a single style of *pro-forma* application form for multi-centre[2] research of that kind. We recommended the adoption of exactly this measure in our Report to the Department of Health in 1992. A single standardised *pro-forma* would overcome a serious cause of delay and inefficiency in the review of multi-centre research, namely the duplication of effort involved in approaching different application procedures for each relevant REC. As we shall see in Chapter Twelve, some of the current delays in the review process produce quite indefensible obstacles to the development and hence the provision of new medicines and other treatments; the multiplicity of *pro-formas* is one cause of these delays, and there seems only what we might call a diplomatic case against the adoption of a standard form. This case, resting on little more than the resistance of individual RECs to an acknowledgment of the rôle and competence of their colleagues elsewhere, seems to us to be insupportable in the face of the gains in effectiveness and efficiency offered by a single form.

If such a form were developed satisfactorily such that it met the requirements we have specified here, then the logical thing to do would be to adopt it generally for all protocol applications. It's true that most multi-centre research concerns pharmaceutical trials, and so one might think that a specially restricted, standardised form could be reserved simply for multi-centre research and that the case for a standard general *pro-forma* has not been made. But there are indeed other kinds of multi-centre research which would benefit from standard application forms even more substantially, if anything, than would pharmaceutical research, owing to the larger numbers of centres typically involved; public health and epidemiology studies are common examples. The large-scale randomised controlled trial is still the 'gold standard' in current scientific clinical research, and if the need for the routine formal assessment of new technology and techniques were generally recognised, then the multi-location model would readily extend to that assessment. A standardised *pro-forma* that accommodated these kinds of research would surely also accommodate the kinds of local, single-centre research that make up the rest of an REC's workload. In itself it would not ensure a uniformly high standard of ethical review, because that is finally the responsibility of REC members: but it would help considerably towards general standards of effective and efficient preparation for members' deliberations and it would stimulate higher standards in researchers' construction of their protocols.

Notes

1   Doyal, L., 'Towards a standard application form for LRECs', *Bulletin of Medical Ethics*, 101 (1994), pp. 15-28.

2   We will subsequently use the term 'multi-location', for reasons that will be discussed in Chapter Twelve.

Chapter Ten

Ethical review and the law

10.1 The absence of statutory requirement in the United Kingdom

It is stipulated in most leases that we should paint our houses outside every three years and inside every seven years, but no-one ever thinks of doing up a school teacher.
(H.G.Wells)

It would be too large an undertaking for this book to deal with the law in all the jurisdictions relevant to ethical review. The largest such jurisdiction, that of the United States, has fairly recently been comprehensively dealt with by Levine[1]. The law in European countries is in some ways a rather fluid phenomenon since the various Directives issued at European Union level seem to be adopted by the relevant countries at different rates[2]. However, it seems to us that the jurisdiction with which we are familiar will in any case serve well enough to illustrate the general issues that would be important from the point of view of REC members anywhere. Accordingly, in this chapter we shall be concerned with the situation which obtains in the United Kingdom and more specifically to the law in England and Wales, Scottish law being in many respects different. (Our shorthand references below to 'U.K. law' or to 'British law' should be taken to mean the law in England and Wales.) Where the actual legal situation is different in other jurisdictions, nevertheless the relevant considerations seem to us still to apply in considering the value of any particular legal solution.

Neither a system of ethical review nor the winning of ethical approval is a statutory requirement for carrying out clinical research in the United Kingdom, nor is there any indication that this situation is likely to change in the near future. Some commentators, for instance Montgomery, partly explain this by suggesting that in effect all those powers which the Secretary of State might need to enforce ethical review are already held in existing law[3]. There is, Montgomery argues, a power to enforce the general provision for ethical review on the part of a Health Authority, in terms of the requirements upon Health Authorities to conform to certain relationships between themselves and the Department of Health, and this gives effective statutory force to many apparently merely advisory documents, of which the Department of Health's *Guidelines* is one. So, for instance, current National Health Service (NHS) employment contracts can compel NHS staff to submit their research proposals to an REC; employment law in England and Wales, according to Montgomery, provides for the enforceability of detailed aspects of such contracts. Whether this precise argument extends to private researchers who use NHS patients as subjects is debatable; it is more likely that research could as a matter of fact not be carried out on NHS patients without the active cooperation of at least some contracted employee of the NHS, so that in practice the contractual restrictions on NHS staff could effectively prevent authorisation of the use of NHS patients in any private research that had not as a matter of fact been put before an ethics committee.

There are four further practical, non-legislative kinds of restraint which might to some extent forestall the need for statutory enforcement of ethical review processes.   First, the specifications of good clinical practice have become increasingly formalised and uniform at an international level. For instance within Europe, the Committee on Proprietary Medicinal Products guidance requires and specifies not merely the fact but the content of ethical review[4].   Second, some licensing regulations such as those of the United States Food and Drug Administration specifically require licensees to have obtained ethical approval for the relevant products; this applies to anyone wishing to market products in the United States, and it covers all research associated with those products wherever it may be conducted.   Third, the U.K. Medicines Control Agency has rules restricting the improper use of substances in research. A Clinical Trials Certificate or a Clinical Trials Exemption Certificate must be obtained by anyone wishing to test relevant substances in clinical research. Such certificates are obtained prior to receiving ethical approval (and RECs generally insist on seeing documentation which confirms the issue of the certificates before ethical approval will be granted); this means of course that the certificates don't in themselves guarantee submission to the subsequent full ethical review procedure, but the certificates do express a rudimentary and preliminary check on what is done in research.   Fourth, most reputable academic journals nowadays require contributing authors to have obtained ethical approval for any clinical research whose results they wish to publish or report in those journals. (Given the current career pressures on clinicians to research and to publish, it is probably not too cynical to imagine that this last requirement constitutes as effective a constraint as any on the majority of researchers working within the National Health Service.) In practice, therefore, it is difficult for individual researchers to conduct any substantial clinical research on human subjects without reference to the processes of ethical review. The fact that a determined dissenter can evade virtually any reasonable system of regulation applies, of course, to statutory regulation more or less as much as it does to voluntary or informal regulation. It might seem that the case for adding a specific statutory requirement to the existing practical requirements has not been made.

There are, however, arguments that can be put forward, largely concerning what we might call the symbolic or 'declaratory' role of the law[5]. Such an argument might begin by asking: what signals do we send by withholding statutory status from ethical review? Are we not advertising the regrettable impression that in the United Kingdom we take ethical review and therefore ethical conduct of clinical research less seriously than many other things which are subject to the law, for instance the hours of shop opening, or the regulation of gambling? The argument might go on to claim that British research facilities will inevitably enjoy the wrong kind of image on the international research arena, so that multinational research sponsors will regard British patients as less well protected than their American counterparts, for instance. The disadvantages of such an image concern, first, British patients, who might be thought by some less scrupulous research sponsors to be more readily available as subjects in dubious research; and second, they concern also British researchers and research facilities, in that the more scrupulous research sponsors might prefer to fund research elsewhere, in institutions which **are** subject to the *imprimatur* of statutory ethical review, when it comes to demonstrating that they have satisfied the requirements of export and distribution of their resulting products to the lucrative American market. (As against this view, we have heard it complained that some pharmaceutical research activity has been diverted from Britain as a result of delays in the cumbersome review process for multi-location research – to be discussed in Chapter Twelve – suggesting that the situation is more complicated than a matter simply of image[6].)

10.2   Animals, human subjects and legal protections

> *There was one poor tiger that hadn't got a Christian.*
> (Punch)

The image of under-protection seems initially to be reinforced when the absence of statutory protection for human research subjects is contrasted with the long standing legal protection of animal research subjects in the United Kingdom[7]. One often hears the ironic comment that Britain is so much a nation of animal lovers that it offers better protection to animals than it does to humans when it comes to clinical experimentation.

Of course this argument begs several questions, not least the question of whether it is even remotely true that animals fare better than humans. A sizeable and vocal constituency of opinion in favour of 'animal rights' and of putting an end to vivisection and other animal experimentation practices is convinced that it is certainly not remotely true!   One does not need to be a member of such organisations to recognise that the so-called LD50 tests, which establish what dosage of a substance will cause the deaths of only half the individuals who receive it, are not performed on human subjects. And for once we don't need to add the rider 'At least, not officially' to the observation. Ample legal powers already exist, under a range of categories from criminal negligence and battery at one end to manslaughter, attempted murder and murder itself at the other, to prevent human research subjects being treated like animals. Indeed, one of the things that the defenders of 'animal rights' complain of is that the preliminary studies of toxicity, mutagenicity and teratology in new substances intended for use in humans are indeed carried out, not in humans but in animals. Those who are sceptical of 'animal rights' will of course be heartily relieved that things are done in this order; even animal sympathisers are usually reluctant to suggest that the initial toxicity tests should be done in humans.

The ironic claim above begs another obvious question: this is the question of whether, if one wants to secure ethically appropriate standards of protection for human subjects, the law is either necessary or sufficient. The defenders of 'animal rights' can make a strong case for suggesting that an uncritical reliance on the law cannot be sufficient, because usually the law will simply prescribe limits which are set by a moral debate that takes place prior to the law. The law generally reflects existing, conventional moral views. So the campaign for greater protection for animal subjects is first and foremost a campaign for the moral high ground from which, campaigners suppose, existing laws will be seen to be hopelessly inadequate: only when (indeed, if) that high ground is captured can laws follow that will satisfy the proponents of 'animal rights'.

Next, and recalling that the present system of ethical review does not enjoy statutory foundations, the question of whether further law is even necessary for proper protection of human research subjects falls back upon the prior question of whether the present system manages to offer proper protection. The present system can be seen as a mixture of criminal laws covering physical mistreatment of persons (relevant to a huge range of contexts inside and outside the clinical arena, of course) and a semi-voluntary system for ethical reflection on new research proposals. If the REC system works as it is meant to, then the case for bringing in further legal protections has not been made. Remember that in the previous section, the case we considered in favour of statutory requirement did not seriously rely on the actual so much as the perceived protection of British research subjects. If the REC system does not work as it is meant to, then the shortcomings must be identified before we can prescribe a remedy. The bringing in of new laws might be necessary if the problem were that the present requirements of ethical review were regularly flouted by a cavalier research community. But there seems to be no evidence that this is now the case. Until we can be confident that RECs uniformly work to a high standard of effectiveness and efficiency, with the benefits of a wide range of experienced, articulate and well prepared members, we cannot simply blame the shortcomings of the system on its lack of statutory establishment.

Interestingly, this does in itself suggest another possible argument for statutory establishment of ethical review. It might be argued that a suitable law is necessary in order to force the hand of the appropriate administrative authorities in making available proper provision, resourcing and training for fully functional RECs. We have already noted that under-resourcing is a chronic, widespread and seriously debilitating problem for the provision of effective ethical review. Unfortunately there are no good grounds for thinking that the answer to this lies in statutory regulation, for the simple reason that if the political will exists to make these resources available then they will be made available by the mechanisms of health policy; and if the political will does not exist, then no law which substantively compelled those sorts of resources will be enacted. However, those who are attracted by the argument concerning the 'signalling' effect of statutory requirement might also think that there is something to be said for pursuing statutory regulation, as a means to forcing the issue of proper resourcing of ethical review onto the political agenda – making resources for ethical review the subject of a public debate. The presence or otherwise of the necessary political will would at least be made visible, and the unwillingness to provide resources for effective ethical review would have to be defended rather more publicly than hitherto.

The question of legal protection of human research subjects is of course more than a matter of the prior scrutiny of research: it is a matter also of what happens to them in the course of the research actually being carried out, and indeed subsequent to it. In particular, the question arises as to what legal protections human research subjects enjoy in the event that they suffer unforeseen harms. We shall examine this question next.

10.3   Negligence, non-negligent harms and subject indemnity

> *...any story against another woman is instantly*
> *believed, even on the flimsiest evidence.*
> (Bertrand Russell)

The results of conducting clinical research on human subjects can sometimes be very unfortunate – however remote, there is always the possibility that an unforeseen and serious harm will befall a research subject. In that unhappy event, the subject will naturally want to be compensated, and may well wish to use the law, if necessary, in order to obtain that compensation.

We can make a basic division of the possibility of such harm, into two general sorts of circumstances: those that involve negligence, and those that do not. And we can further divide the question of negligence, giving separate consideration to, on the one hand, negligent practice by a researcher in the performance of otherwise acceptable research, and on the other hand negligent practice by an REC in terms of careless or otherwise unacceptable conduct in giving ethical approval to research which should not have received such approval and which was ethically unacceptable. We shall consider the question of negligent practice by the REC in the next section, concerning the legal responsibilities of RECs and their members.

First, then, let us consider negligent practice in the actual conduct of research. Working on the assumption that the research protocol in question is otherwise ethically sound, then we can deal fairly summarily with this form of negligence, since the REC's responsibilities in this matter are limited. The REC should, as part of conducting ethical review in a responsible manner, be satisfied that the particular researcher is herself a responsible person, fitted to carry out the research for which she is seeking ethical approval. Beyond this, the REC has a rather vague responsibility to monitor the progress of research; but as we saw in section 8.6 this responsibility has not been clearly spelled out and presently relies either on the integrity of the researcher, in drawing adverse events to the committee's attention, or on discovering information through a third-party report, largely by chance. Clearly the REC should act on any information which it does receive and which leads it to suppose that the researcher may have been negligent. However, the REC's role in **forestalling** negligent action by the researcher is more or less confined to the review process itself.

Research subjects who have been harmed as a result of what they consider negligence by the researcher face the task of establishing that negligence to the law's satisfaction. This is no easy matter, requiring the subject to show that the harm that befell him should have been – but was not – foreseen by the researcher, or that the researcher deliberately withheld information from him, or otherwise misled him, in obtaining his consent to take part. This is traditionally very difficult to establish in British law, and threatens to leave an injured research subject in a near-impossible position – namely that of having suffered a (possibly) serious harm whilst being unable to obtain compensation because of the problem of demonstrating negligence. In addition, of course, subjects who were harmed as a result of simple misfortune or unforeseeable events could not appeal to the law in terms of negligence. For these reasons, it is important that research subjects also be protected against non-negligent harm, by being given legally binding assurances of compensation on the part of the sponsoring institution; this will usually be a commercial company in the case of pharmaceutical research. It is to say the least unclear whether subjects can hope for as much in the case of research conducted entirely under the aegis of the National Health Service, without external sponsors. There is no central indemnity provided or funded at the level of the Department of Health; responsibility is left to the health commissioning authorities or trusts who actually employ the researchers in question[8]. The really crucial point about any compensation for non-negligent harms is that it must be available to the research subject without going to law, and certainly without having to prove to the satisfaction of the law that negligence has occurred. This sort of assurance is referred to generally as indemnity; and it is a key feature of any ethically sound research protocol that it clearly and unambiguously commits the sponsoring institution to providing indemnity against non-negligent harms which might arise from taking part in the research. In Britain, pharmaceutical companies typically offer a standard form of indemnity set out in the Guidelines of the Association of British Pharmaceutical Industry (ABPI), and this is specified in the information given to research subjects. It excludes liability in cases where there has been negligence on the part of the subject himself, or 'wrongful action' by a third party such as a doctor[9]. Initially, this makes it look as though if a harm were to occur it would place the unfortunate claimant in a kind of double jeopardy, having to prove negligence to obtain compensation through the courts, but having to prove the absence of negligence to obtain compensation through the indemnity scheme! In practice the onus of demonstrating negligence on the part of the researcher or other carers now falls on the indemnifier, who will be expected either to pay the compensation straightforwardly **or**, in seeking to avoid this, to demonstrate negligence to the satisfaction of the courts – thus paving the way for the claimant to receive compensation in law. The ABPI scheme advises that compensation should proceed anyway if negligence were alleged against the pharmaceutical company involved.

It is reassuring to see the British pharmaceutical industry taking non-negligent indemnity as seriously as they presently do. In fact their doing so has the effect of showing up the failings of others, in the light of which we can see a serious inequity of treatment between those who are the subjects of pharmaceutical research sponsored by the pharmaceutical industry, and those who are the subjects of other kinds of clinical research funded by other sponsors. This second, probably much larger, group can presently have no general expectations of non-negligent cover. The situation is at best patchy, with some sponsors (including some Hospital Trusts) offering cover that is underwritten by insurance agreements, and other sponsors offering no such thing. Perhaps most strikingly of all, they are simply not required to offer cover by the current Department of Health *Guidelines*. This is a serious injustice to patient research subjects in the United Kingdom. Only relatively recently have patients gained one particular public health protection which had previously been denied them; hospital establishments have lost their Crown immunity from prosecution. Before this happened, patients suffering illness and damage caused by the transmission of disease through, for example, food prepared in dirty kitchens, were not protected by public health legislation in the same way as people who bought food in restaurants. Restaurant owners were all along subject to the sanctions of environmental health legislation. Now this protection has been extended to all patients in hospital, and the hospital authorities are subject to precisely the same conditions as outside establishments. Yet in the area of clinical research, where health damage may result directly from the participation of patients in trials, those subjects in National Health Service-sponsored research may be denied the protections they would enjoy if the research were sponsored by pharmaceutical companies. There is no moral justification for this anomaly.

RECs should be able to insist that all research which carries even minimal risk of harm to the subject – and this effectively means all research which involves clinical contact of any more significant kind than merely conducting interviews or questionnaires – have as an integral part of the protocol a proper undertaking of indemnity against non-negligent harm. This undertaking should also be a part of the subject information sheet and the subject consent form (see section 6.5 above). But in Britain some centrally funded research does not ordinarily carry such indemnity. The question then arises as to whether the REC can approve otherwise acceptable research that doesn't offer its subjects this protection. Tempting though it is to take a 'hard' line on this point and make such indemnity a qualifying condition for ethical approval, we must nonetheless recall that doing so would at present halt much valuable research in its tracks, and that the problem is to a limited extent approached through ensuring that subjects are recruited only on the basis of a full understanding of their vulnerability in the event of a non-negligent harm. (Utilitarians can't help on this question: the greatest long-term benefit might be obtained by tolerating unsatisfactory indemnity arrangements in the interests of permitting otherwise high quality research to proceed; but it might instead come from obstructing such research and forcing the issue of centrally funded indemnity upon an unwilling Government.) The best that can presently be said is that RECs must take this decision in the light of the balance of risks and benefits accruing to any particular non-indemnified research.

10.4   The legal responsibilities of RECs and their members

We find for the defendant, much as we dislike him.
(A.P. Herbert)

We must now consider what is legally required for the REC to carry out its duties responsibly. We have already noted that the DoH *Guidelines* emphasise that the REC must always be able to show that it has acted reasonably in reaching its decisions. The trouble is that 'acting reasonably' is a rather vague notion. One commentator, Morgan, notes that English law has no absolute standard of perfect or even of adequate practice – after all, the methods and working practices of different committees will vary and it will be hard to specify a standard to which they should all conform[10].

On the other hand it is clearly important that during its discussions the REC takes into account all the features of a protocol, and of the local situation, which could reasonably be thought relevant – and it is just as important that irrelevant matters, leading perhaps to bias or prejudice, are kept out of account. Among the relevant factors, of course, is the adequacy of the information given to the subject, and on which his consent is based. The REC will want to be satisfied that all those risks which are inherent in the research should be formally and properly explained to the research subject prior to his giving consent – as well, of course, as being satisfied that the risks in question are not so serious as to disqualify the research from receiving ethical approval (see Chapter Five). Beyond these matters, any personal interests that might dispose members to judge one way or another should always be openly declared and properly minuted. In some circumstances these interests might disqualify a particular member from adjudicating on that particular protocol, and hence the member should withdraw, and the withdrawal should be minuted. If all these things are done, then it would be difficult to regard an REC's judgement as having been negligent in law.

Moreover, in the UK it is extremely unlikely that an REC or its members would ever have to demonstrate the propriety of their actions before the law. Members of RECs are ordinarily protected from any liability arising from their actions, by either of two sources of indemnity: National Health Service (NHS) employees enjoy NHS indemnity; members who are not NHS employees should receive an undertaking of indemnity from the Health Authority to which the REC is responsible. The Department of Health's *Guidelines* specifically require the Health Authority concerned to bear all the costs arising out of such a member's performance of his duties – and to give the member an undertaking to that effect – unless gross lack of care or misconduct on the part of the member can be shown[11]. Again of course it is not easy to specify when such misconduct could be thought to arise or be proven against an REC member. It seems to be generally agreed that a member who acts in good faith, declares any relevant interests, and takes into account in his judgements those things which could reasonably be thought to be relevant, will be held to have acted properly. Even where it was supposed that an REC member had not acted properly in this way, Morgan suggests that the only real likelihood of facing a legal suit would be where a member had a personal professional liability insurance cover; those insurers might contest any attempt on the part of the Health Authority to recover from them costs which the Health Authority had borne, arising out of genuinely negligent conduct on the part of the member concerned[12]. But the likelihood is remote, and the Department of Health's *Guidelines* themselves note that:

> there is little prospect of a successful claim against an LREC member for a mishap arising from research approved as ethical by the LREC. Any such claim would lie principally against the researcher concerned, and against the NHS body under the auspices of which the research took place. The principal defendants should seek to have any claim against an LREC member struck out.[13]

10.5   Some statutory exceptions

> *I shall be an autocrat: that's my trade. And*
> *the good Lord will forgive me: that's His.*
> (Empress Catherine the Great)

We noted at the outset of this chapter that ethical review has no statutory basis in the United Kingdom. However, whilst this general situation may be unlikely to change soon, there are already some interesting exceptions to it, and we may usefully mention them before passing on from questions of the law.

The exceptions are twofold. The first concerns a specific field of clinical practice, a field which is inherently so experimental that the distinction between research and practice tends to break down. Certain medical techniques in the field of assisted reproduction involve research upon, or manipulation of, human embryos, and these can be carried out only in centres that are licensed by the Human Fertilisation and Embryo Authority (HFEA), whose requirements include that such treatment will be approved by an ethics committee, which may be an ethics committee set up at the clinical centre concerned[14]. The HFEA is a statutory authority established by an Act of Parliament and its requirements carry the force of law[15]; furthermore, owing to the blurred distinction between research and practice in this area, it could reasonably be argued that their requirements represent a legal obligation to conduct ethical review of at least some clinical research. We will pursue this a little further in Chapter Thirteen.

(The UK position is less clear in two other clinical fields: much genetic medicine is clearly experimental, but the Clothier Report's requirement that research and practice in this field be submitted to an appropriate ethics committee lacks the legal enforceability which the HFEA's requirements enjoy. On the other hand, the statutory Unrelated Live Transplants Regulatory Authority (ULTRA), which formally approves applications for organ transplants from living donors who are not close relatives of the recipient, is concerned essentially with an established clinical practice that could not any longer really be regarded as a research activity.)

The second formal exception to the general non-statutory situation of ethical review comes from a European Commission Directive which the United Kingdom was obliged to implement as from 1st of January 1992[16]. This Directive laid down certain documentary requirements in connection with applications for product licences (and thus for marketing permission) for new medicines. These requirements, like those of the specification of good clinical practice to which we referred at the outset, include the stipulation that protocols for clinical trials must be submitted by the sponsor and/or the investigator to the relevant ethics committee, and that the committee's approval must be obtained in writing before the trials begin. This is potentially very far-reaching, especially in view of the large proportion of research connected with the development of new drugs.

Be that as it may, the present system of ethical review does nonetheless lack any overall statutory basis. However, this is obviously no ground for complacency or casualness on the part of either researchers or sponsors in submitting protocols for review, or on the part of RECs themselves in carrying out that review. The law is often brought in as a way of defending interests or concerns that are essentially moral in character, but which are nonetheless not sufficiently respected in practice. Ethical review of research is inherently and by definition a moral concern, and thus carries its own compelling reason for being done properly. It would be only if the present informal (and to some small extent voluntary) system proved ultimately incapable of doing the job properly that there would really be a need for specific laws. At the end of the day, then, the challenge is to make ethical review effective and efficient; therefore the question of whether a statutory basis is really necessary for ethical review is secondary to the question of whether we can make the present system work. And it is with that question that this book is overwhelmingly concerned.

Notes

1   Levine, R., *Ethics and Regulation of Clinical Research*, Baltimore and Munich: Urban & Schwarzenberg (1986).

2   For instance it is not clear that the United Kingdom had substantially implemented European Commission Directive No. 91/507/EEC at the required effective date of 1st January 1992.

3   Montgomery, J, 'New law not needed for better RECs', *Bulletin of Medical Ethics*, 78 (1992), pp. 34-5.

4   Working Party on Efficacy of Medicinal Products, Commission of the European Communities, *Good Clinical Practice for Trials on Medicinal Products in the European Community*, Brussels: Committee on Proprietary Medicinal Products, Document 111/2976/88-EN (1991). For a discussion of its implications, see Scott, G. and Goode, K., 'Reporting the outcome of ethics

review', *Bulletin of Medical Ethics*, 110 (1995), pp. 16-17.

5   See for instance Neuberger, J., *Ethics and Health Care: the Role of Research Ethics Committees in the United Kingdom*, London: King's Fund Institute (1992), p.45.

6   Dr. Frank Wells of the Association of British Pharmaceutical Industries, oral report to the Ethical Review Training Conference, Robinson College, Cambridge, September 1994.

7   The world's first law on the matter was passed in England and Wales under the Cruelty to Animals Act of 1876; see Hampson, J., 'Legislation and the changing consensus' in Langley, G. (ed.), *Animal Experimentation: the Consensus Changes*, Basingstoke: Macmillan (1989), pp. 219-51.

8   One health care Trust known to the authors routinely specifies in its information and consent forms to research subjects that they need not establish negligence in order to **submit** a claim; however, those who read further discover that it is only in the event that negligence is proved that claimants can expect their claim to **succeed**.

9   Association of British Pharmaceutical Industries (ABPI), *Clinical Trial Compensation Guidelines*, London: ABPI (1991). This document treats healthy volunteers and patients as separate groups, and separate provisions apply to each.

10   Morgan, D., 'An introduction to legal aspects of ethical review' in Evans, D., Evans, M., Greaves, D. and Morgan, D., *Trainers' Manual for the Training of Members of Research Ethics Committees*, (Annexe to Report to the Department of Health on the training of REC members), Swansea: Centre for Philosophy and Health Care (1992), p. 6.10.

11   Department of Health, *Local Research Ethics Committees*, London: Department of Health, para. 2.11.

12   Morgan, *op. cit.*, p 6.9.

13   Department of Health, *loc. cit.*

14   Human Fertilisation and Embryology Authority, *Code of Practice*, London: Human Fertilisation and Embryology Authority (1993, revised) paras. 9.6, 9.7.

15   Morgan, D. & Lee, R.G., *Blackstone's Guide to the Human Fertilisation and Embryology Act 1990*, London: Blackstone Press (1991), especially Chapters 1 and 4.

16   European Commission Directive No. 91/507/EEC, dated 19th July 1991.

Chapter Eleven

Why local? The importance of variable circumstances

11.1   The Committee and its 'patch'

Whaur's yer Wully Shakespeare noo?
(Anonymous Scottish theatregoer)

The pattern in the United Kingdom of distinguishing Research Ethics Committees in terms of the geographical location for which they are broadly responsible is perhaps more historical than the result of a deliberate policy. It would be natural for research-minded institutions to seek conveniently available guidance when ethical considerations first became important in the way that specific research was conceived and proposed. As well as consulting senior colleagues through the various professional bodies such as medical Royal Colleges, it would be straightforward for researchers to gain ethical clearance from discussing their plans with colleagues locally.

The Department of Health *Guidelines* give no compelling rationale for local ethical review; rather they work on the basis of the situation as it is presently found. Indeed whilst the resource and financial implications of specific research projects are recognised to be a matter for local management, the *Guidelines* actually specify ethical review as needing to be independent of local management[1]. The *Guidelines* refer to the 'convenience' of locally organised ethical review but note also that RECs exist 'to advise any NHS body' and there is no requirement that the advice must be local to the body being advised. However,, it seems clear that some very good reasons can be given for the geographical relationship between an REC and its 'patch' – normally a National Health Service district. Some aspects of research, particularly research needing generalisable conclusions, aim at being independent of considerations about where the research is actually carried out – these of course are the aspects of scientific validity and repeatability. But the very aspects that most concern the REC, namely the ethical questions arising out of how subjects will be treated, are as much tied to the particular circumstances of who will conduct the research, on whom and where, as they are tied to 'good science'.

11.2   Personal knowledge of researchers and facilities

I wasn't kissing her. I was whispering in her mouth.
(Chico Marx)

A Committee which knows at first hand who will carry out a particular piece of research, and with what facilities and on what premises, can judge the standards of care and safety applicable to its research subjects in a way that no other Committee can.   Furthermore, that Committee will be able to advise and assist the researcher over a long period in optimising the design and conduct of her research as far as it concerns the well-being of the research subjects.   It will be able to encourage the completion of clear, accurate and informative *pro forma* application forms at the first time of asking, rather than by means of repeated submissions, thereby reducing the time wasted on the part of researcher and Committee alike.

The Committee will also be able to conduct more direct and more effective interviews with those researchers of whose work it has experience, knowing how much research they have taken on, how sensitively they have recruited subjects in the past, how successful they have been in completing previous research and so on. It will also be able to judge more accurately when an interview is necessary and when it is not – again, saving time for both Committee and researcher. Finally, an important but easily overlooked point is made by Levine who observes that a local Committee is known to the researchers themselves, and can take responsibility for its own decisions, including decisions which researchers might find frustrating or disappointing[2]. The local Committee is on hand to explain its reasons directly, and can help the researchers' appreciation of and respect for the reasons on which its decisions are based, an outcome which should lead to the submission of better-designed research in the future.

11.3   Local knowledge of subject populations

There are still parts of Wales where the only
concession to gaiety is a striped shroud.
(Gwyn Thomas)

A certain amount of research, particularly involving detailed questionnaires concerning personal and social circumstances, will from time to time need to be considered in terms of its effect on the sensitivities of certain population groups, particularly subjects from specific ethnic or religious groups.   Occasionally such research will be quite inappropriate;   for instance to ignore Islamic sensitivities concerning frank questioning about sexual behaviour patterns could lead a researcher into giving great offence even at the stage of recruiting prospective subjects.   It falls to the REC to judge whether this is true of any given research, precisely because the REC can have knowledge of local demographic features that would not be known by a more remote committee (such as those frequently attached to central funding bodies sponsoring medical and social research). Since locally-based researchers as well could also reasonably be expected to have such knowledge, so it is more likely that problems of this sort will occur in connection with large scale multi-location studies designed by researchers based elsewhere, perhaps most usually studies in epidemiological or public health research involving the prospective use of questionnaires.

Local knowledge of subject populations can be important in other ways too: the REC should be well placed to know whether, for instance, a particular patient group in its own locality has in recent months been exposed to several pieces of research, making additional research inappropriate, insensitive or even clinically hazardous within too narrow a period of time;   multiple concurrent studies of respiratory or digestive diseases might be coordinated to avoid the problems of repeated X-ray or endoscopic examination – but they might not.   Again it is the REC on the spot who can determine this.   Whilst of course such cases ought to be picked up by good exclusion criteria, the REC may be able to see immediately from a protocol that very many potential subjects in their own locality are likely to fall foul of a particular exclusion criterion, thus making the proposed research simply impractical.

Lastly, local sensitivities may be particularly sharpened by some recent event which might well not be known either to a distant researcher or to a central research ethics committee, remote from the locality concerned;   industrial accidents, environmental dangers, or other socially painful events may have occurred sufficiently recently to make specific research proposals quite inappropriate in a particular locality, and it is more realistic to expect this to be noticed and responded to by a local Committee.   Some kinds of research are obviously especially vulnerable to conflicts of this kind;   for instance a multi-location study attempting to compare the reliability of diagnostic methods in cases of child sexual abuse could obviously provoke strong local hostility in the aftermath of highly publicised and controversial criminal investigations. Whilst local researchers might be relied upon to realise this and to decline the opportunity to take part, the REC is the public's guarantee of sensitivity and discretion.

11.4   The task of monitoring research

Fierce cannonade from Italian ships. No casualties.
(Signal from besieged Austrian defenders at Lissa)

We have already noted that the REC's rôle officially extends to monitoring local on-going research, and to intervening to stop research when necessary. There are various possible ways in which the monitoring might be done:

- site inspections before and after approval, particularly in the case of researchers or facilities not previously known to the Committee, to enable the Committee to be satisfied that the means really exist to supply the safeguards which have been promised. Single-centre research may be most pertinent here, or multi-centre research where the sponsoring company lacks a proven record of satisfying itself regarding the ability of the local researcher to meet the centrally-specified criteria;

- requiring a mid-term interim report to be submitted by the researcher for evaluation by the Committee, particularly as regards the notification of any adverse events or the withdrawal of subjects from the research, the reasons in each case to be stipulated;

- scrutiny of the actual consent process, presumably including inspection of specimens of signed consents: for this not to be meaningless, some mechanism would have to be found for ensuring that the REC had access to a genuinely representative (probably random) sample of these, and could if necessary interview subjects under suitable conditions;

- requiring the regular submission of interim reports at six-monthly intervals; these need not be elaborate documents but should certainly indicate the progress of the research including the starting date – far too many research projects obtain ethical approval (and thus occupy the review process) without ever actually being executed. Additionally they should obviously notify the REC of any relevant early indications, including adverse events, which bear upon the interests of the research subjects;

- requiring the submission of final reports, including copies of reports submitted to sponsors, and copies of manuscripts submitted for publication, together with documentary evidence regarding the details of submission; backing this up perhaps in appropriate cases with a requirement to know the outcome of research submissions, and to receive copies of the referees' reports on the manuscripts;

- requiring copies of any resultant publication.

The resource and time implications of any of these measures are obvious – they are huge, and most RECs already find it difficult to discharge their functions simply in terms of review. Nonetheless, can ethical review be meaningful in the absence of monitoring and follow-up? The question arises, therefore, of whether the Health Authority (to put the matter once again in its British context) has an obligation to provide its own, perhaps more efficient, channels for this kind of monitoring, reporting to the REC for the Committee's follow-up review (the REC subsequently reporting in turn to the Health Authority). Obviously we cannot settle such questions here; our present point is simply to acknowledge that within the current ethical review structure it is to the local REC that this responsibility falls. But clearly the local knowledge held by the REC concerning its 'patch' makes the REC the appropriate body to oversee the monitoring of research and to re-assess ethical approval of particular research projects in the light of monitoring.

11.5   Local responses to 'central' ethical approval

> *He trusted neither of them as far as he could spit, and he*
> *was a poor spitter, lacking both distance and control.*
> (P.G. Wodehouse)

As we shall see in the consideration of multi-location research in the next chapter, RECs may often be asked to scrutinise research proposals which are advertised as having satisfied some more central ethical committee such as a research ethics committee set up by a funding body (such as the Medical Research Council) or by a professional body (such as the medical Royal Colleges). RECs' reactions to this situation provoke (and illuminate) questions of what their relative rôles should be *vis-à-vis* more centralised bodies, most particularly in reviewing research being conducted simultaneously in several areas. The next chapter will be devoted entirely to tackling those questions; but it would be helpful here to set out a guiding principle that will underpin that discussion.

The principle is this: that there are effectively two distinct sets of questions arising when we consider any new proposed research. First, there is the consideration of the **protocol as such** which embodies the scientific conception and design of the proposed research as well as its general ethical characteristics; then second, if the protocol as such is satisfactory there is the consideration of **implementing the research locally**. The two stages need not constitute watertight separate discussions, and certainly the second must make continual reference to the first, but we believe the review of any research proposal can be modelled like this. In effect, the first stage involves our asking whether the proposed research is a good idea in general; the second involves our asking whether, even if so, it would be a good idea to carry it out in this particular location, on this particular patient population, under the control of these particular researchers.

All of these questions are properly in mind in the REC's discussion, and it's logical to pursue them in this order. The second stage really explores the questions that the first stage puts on one side: deciding whether the protocol as such is any good is a general question of principle. But if (and only if) the requirements in principle are satisfied, and the research is such that it could be carried out appropriately, then the REC must go on to ask whether that is likely on its own patch, under the circumstances envisaged locally. Now it is clear that whereas any competent central committee could consider the protocol as such, only the local REC on the spot can tackle the second set of questions – which are, in effect, those that we have been identifying and emphasising throughout this chapter. The irreducible rôle for the local REC, in any review process where a central body has already approved a piece of research in principle, is to ask whether it is a good idea that the research be implemented in the local context.

Finally, the REC may have one further job that could not be undertaken more centrally: dealing with the surprise, frustration or disappointment of local researchers who thought that central approval would be decisive.   Levine sensibly observes that in order to reserve judgement with authority and credibility, the local REC must have established its own independence in the minds of local researchers, and needs researchers to appreciate that its decisions are locally important because they are locally arrived at[3].

This 'division of labour' sounds simple enough. However, the problems to which we believe it contributes a solution have been historically somewhat intractable. To these we shall turn in the next chapter.

Notes

1   Department of Health, *Local Research Ethics Committees*, London: Department of Health (1991), para. 1.1.

2   Levine, R., *Ethics and Regulation of Clinical Research*, Baltimore & Munich: Urban & Schwarzenberg (1986), pp. 342-3.

3   Levine, R., *op. cit.*, p. 343.

Chapter Twelve

The special challenge of
multi-location research

12.1   Defining multi-location research

May I ask what you were hoping to see out of a Torquay bedroom window?
Sydney Opera House, perhaps? The Hanging Gardens of Babylon?
(John Cleese and Connie Booth, as rasped by Basil Fawlty)

In early 1992 we were commissioned by the Department of Health to study the problems involved in conducting ethical review of multi-centre clinical research. As soon as we began to consult researchers about the matter it became obvious that there was a good deal of unclarity about the meaning of 'multi-centre research'. To begin with, was it only multi-centre pharmaceutical trials which faced difficulties from being carried out and hence reviewed in multiple locations? Many researchers impressed upon us that they ran into these difficulties in connection with observational or statistical studies rather than experimental clinical trials, and furthermore that these studies were not conducted in clinical centres so much as in whole districts or geographical areas. Differences like these drew attention to more general differences in methodology which, it was alleged, were often missed by Local Research Ethics Committees in the conduct of their work.

It is generally recognised that many clinical trials need large numbers of subjects. Indeed this is a defining feature of Phase III pharmaceutical research where the reliability and repeatability of the application of a new medicine is under scrutiny. This means that the cohort of research subjects has to be drawn from a large number of geographical areas. Even in much smaller research projects, where relatively rare conditions are being studied it is necessary to spread the net for suitable subjects over a wide area involving numerous clinicians in a variety of locations.

But the range of areas where other kinds of medical-related research is carried out is often much wider than that of most clinical trials. A large proportion of epidemiological and sociological studies are carried out not by resident staff in research centres but by the research staff from a central body (such as the Public Health Laboratory Service) who travel to many districts to make their enquiries. It was suggested to us that such studies should be called multi-district research to distinguish them from clinical trials. Other researchers whom we interviewed were concerned that even this was too narrow a description of the sorts of research which face problems from ethical review of multi-location research. Some such research could indeed be called 'omni-district' research. National risk factor studies, for example, require centrally-based researchers to move quickly into any district where an outbreak of a specific condition has developed and to get detailed answers to their questions before people's memories of the specific circumstances become vague. Often these details may seem to the sufferers themselves to be insignificant. Seeking clearance from local RECs at the time in question would frustrate the exercise and render it futile. It is this kind of research, together with other large-scale epidemiological studies, which runs into the greatest problems of administration and delay in gaining ethical approval, and in order not to lose sight of it we decided to label the research with which we were concerned 'multi-location research' so as to avoid giving unintended prominence to any particular mode of research.

We also came across different views about how many separate locations had to be involved in order to require a distinct system of ethical review. Of those researchers who were concerned about the delays in processing their protocols through the system, most felt that this should be a matter left to the researchers themselves. That is, when the number of committees which must be approached becomes unmanageably large for a given researcher or research team, then the researcher(s) would like to be able to opt into a special, streamlined multi-location system of review. So most studies involving smaller numbers of locations would not need a streamlined system at all. In response to this suggestion, it was put to us that if a new proposed system turned out to be more rigorous than the existing one, then the 'opt-out' would be a means of avoiding the most careful ethical scrutiny; what's more, the mere suspicion of this might prejudice local RECs against those 'opted-out' protocols which they were called on to consider. On balance we thought that there was little weight to this argument. Any new system would need to fight to retain the rigour of the current system whilst also offering improvements in efficiency. Thus we support an informal definition of what constitutes a multi-location research protocol.

12.2　　The trouble with multi-location review

Am in Market Harborough. Where should I be?
(G.K. Chesterton, in a telegram to his wife.)

There have been calls for a streamlining of the ethical review of multi-location clinical research for some time.　These have come largely from clinical researchers and pharmaceutical companies whose interests are clearly threatened by unnecessary delays to the conduct of research.　In March 1992 the UK Department of Health commissioned us to carry out a twelve-week study and report our findings and recommendations to them in May 1992, which we duly did.　Unfortunately the wider consultation which followed turned out to be a very slow process, and it was not until November 1994 that systematic discussions held at the Department of Health began in earnest on the business of reforming ethical review of multi-location research on human subjects.　Those talks are still under way at the time of writing (September 1995);　we will not review the talks as such, but we will review the questions which arose in our original research project on multi-location research review, and which inevitably play a part in the Department's discussions.

We first have to ask whether the purported problems in ethical review of multi-location research (hereafter 'multi-location review') are as serious as has been claimed and whether urgent action is really called for.　In the course of our research we came across various groups of people who were convinced that something had to be done in the short term to correct serious faults in the system. Whilst they shared a good deal of anecdotal evidence with us it was not easy to identify many documented examples of the sorts of delays and weaknesses alleged. We did encounter some serious instances but we had no means of finding out whether or not these represented the tip of an iceberg – as many researchers clearly believed they did.　For example whilst we did find one instance of a clinical trial which had enjoyed the approval of a central ethical review committee, only for that approval later to be withdrawn following the criticism of the protocol by a local committee, we could not predict how many such cases might have occurred if there had been widespread machinery of feedback from local to central committees, thus enabling central approvals to be reconsidered.

Again, the larger the number of committees who have to be consulted, the more difficult is the task of completing the process of review.　This presents a special problem to bodies wishing to carry out public health surveys, such as the Public Health Laboratories Service which ran the listeriosis study cited below, because all areas of the country for which the service is responsible have to be canvassed.　These problems are most typically shared by epidemiologal studies.

By contrast, most multi-location clinical trials concern the fewest possible number of centres consistent with finding enough subjects to produce statistically significant results. This is a somewhat complicated matter, and necessarily beyond the scope of this book. The most we can do here is present an illustrative example. Suppose that in a given period the proportion of patients whose disease remains unchecked even by the best available drugs is 50%. Next, suppose that a new and improved drug is actually able to reduce this figure to 40%, which in relative terms is a one-fifth or 20% gain over the previously-unchecked proportion. Finally, suppose that we want to be able to demonstrate this improvement within the traditional levels of stringency, namely that we shall be 90% confident that the test was actually capable of finding any improvement **and** that there shall be a no greater than 5% risk that the test would exaggerate any improvement. Given all of these requirements, we would actually need to run a clinical trial of 850 patients randomised between the standard treatment and the new treatment[1].

If the actual improvement offered by the new treatment were much greater than this, then obviously fewer patients would be needed in order to demonstrate it: researchers must accordingly have a fair idea of what it is they expect to find before they can design an effective and statistically valid trial to find it. In the present illustration, an improvement of 60% could be detected by a trial involving only 90 patients[2]. For common diseases, even the larger number of patients might over a suitable period be found from perhaps 30 major clinical centres - clearly far fewer than the number of centres involved in public health surveys. In our experience this is typical of multi-location clinical trials. This therefore makes the problems of public health surveys and epidemiological studies rather special and untypical of the whole range of multi-location clinical research.

Of course, this observation does nothing to ease the problems faced by public health and epidemiological researchers and some reform of the system of multi-location review is needed for these categories of research. It might be possible to make exceptional arrangements for these, however, without altering the arrangement for the rest. On balance, however, we are opposed to a marginal solution of this kind, because even though we could not be sure of the scale of the difficulties presented by multi-location review we were still able to pick out serious problems in the system which called for reforms; moreover, the right reforms could encourage more general improvements in ethical review for research on human subjects beyond the category of multi-location research. What then were the problems which we found? We were able to identify two clusters of problems, each of which presented a *prima facie* case for reform of the procedure. The first was the **inefficiency** of the current system and the second the **ineffectivenes** of that system in delivering high quality review.

12.2.1   Inefficiency of multi-location review

A key criterion of efficiency in carrying out multi-location review is the time taken for a given protocol to make its complete passage through the system. Any unjustified delays may squander the investment of research expertise and money and, perhaps more importantly, will impede the progress of medicine and the achievement of higher standards of health care. This can happen in at least the following respects:

Patient care and delays in ethical review

We were informed of one study (whose difficulties have since been documented[3]) where the research was delayed for two years because of the tardiness of some Local Research Ethics Committees in responding and where the cumbersome character of the review process (arising from the multiplicity of REC *pro-forma* application documents as well as from the sheer number of committees to be consulted) may even have resulted in avoidable deaths. It is indeed ironic if the process of ethical review, which is designed to protect the health and interests of vulnerable research subjects, actually results unnecessarily in the deaths of vulnerable patients. In the case of a prevalence study of listeriosis – the worst case which we identified – we also discovered that it took one local REC four months to communicate its approval even after it had made its decision. The earliest possible availability of new and better medicines, diagnostic and therapeutic techniques and increased knowledge of disease conditions is clearly in the interests of all patients and no properly avoidable delay can be justified, even in the name of ethical review. If the actual system of review is itself responsible for unethical outcomes because of its own inefficiency, then such a system cannot be justified or left unreformed.

Commercial patent application times and delays in ethical review

A good deal of pressure is brought to bear on the system of ethical review by the promoters of research both in the form of researchers, whose careers may be advanced by the progress of the research in question, and by sponsoring authorities, who in one way or another want to see the best possible returns for their investment. Perhaps most notable amongst these pressure groups are the pharmaceutical companies who have an obvious interest in expediting ethical review of clinical trials.

It will be useful for us to review the typical history of the discovery, development and marketing of a new medicine in the United Kingdom as the U.K. is one of the top five spending nations on research and development in the innovation of pharmaceutical compounds[4] and is the country which, it is claimed, is subject to the greatest 'squeeze' on the effective patent life of a pharmaceutical product[5]. The effective patent life of a new medicine in the U.K. is calculated as the interval between the U.K. marketing date and the patent expiry date. By the time of our research into the review of multi-centre clinical trials the Centre for Medicines Research had demonstrated that this interval has been compressed owing to the considerable extension of the development phases of new medicines which has occurred since 1960[6], the patents themselves being taken out near the start of the development phase. Whereas in the period 1960-1962 the overall development time was less than four years (including pre-clinical and clinical phases) by 1996 the time is near to eleven years (including the various regulatory hold-ups for Clinical Trials Certificates and product licences). By far the largest growth in development time occurred at the clinical phase of development, the very phase where ethical review becomes necessary. This phase had increased from three to seven years. As a result effective patent life had fallen, it is claimed, from thirteen years in 1960 to less than five years in 1986. Given the vast increase in the cost of developing a new medicine (a cost which has jumped from $7.5 million in the 1950s to $350 million at the present time) and given also the claim made as early as 1982 that by then nineteen years of worldwide sales were required to recover R&D investment in pharmaceutical products[7], the threat to investment in pharmaceutical development of new medicines is considerable. This is exacerbated in the U.K. by the limitations, imposed in the late 1980s by the Government, on drug prescriptions paid for by the National Health Service.

Given this kind of information it would be difficult to resist the view that any further squeeze on the effective patent life of new medicines resulting from avoidable delays in the process of ethical review are unjustifiable. If the system can be streamlined without cost to the research subjects themselves then it ought to be.

Research fatigue and delays in ethical review

As part of our Department of Health research into the conduct of multi-location review we interviewed researchers who conducted large scale multi-location clinical trials. We were told that the scale of the effort required, to chase up local RECs for their adjudications on applications and to respond to the RECs' proposed protocol amendments or to their requests for further information, placed an inordinate burden on the researchers. The main reason for this burden was twofold: it lay in the complexity of the system in which each local REC had its own *pro-forma* application form, and it lay also – we were told – in the the the sheer numbers of those committees. The additional inefficiencies of individual committees simply exacerbated the problems; the underlying difficulty resulted from a system in which such a wide array of committees each required its own separate review process channelled by means of its own separate application documents.

The consequence was that valuable research skills and time were devoted to unnecessary administrative chores, producing weariness in the researchers and a loss of enthusiasm for the research in hand. We were unable to find out what proportion of research projects fell victim to these logistical problems of obtaining ethical approval but were assured that that there were such cases.

The lack of standardised pro-forma *submission documents*

There is a good deal of variety in the ways in which individual local RECs elicit information about submitted protocols from researchers. Most committees have devised their own summary set of questions designed to cover various relevant features of ethical review. Some are much more comprehensive than others. We tried to produce a useful synthesis of a number of such forms which were supplied to us by committees following the distribution of our research Report. It proved to be an impossible task in that any composite *pro-forma* would have been as long as, if not longer than, most protocols we were called upon to review as members of local RECs; for example, one of those presented to us consisted of twenty-six pages of detailed questions. The use of such cumbersome documents would not produce obvious improvements in the speed of ethical review. However, we do think that the production of a standardised *pro-forma* that was universally adopted by all RECs would be of great assistance both to researchers and reviewers of protocols[8,9].

In Chapter Nine we set out the basis for constructing a workable *pro-forma* in terms of the crucial questions to which we think plain language answers are essential for efficient and effective ethical review, and which we think any serious REC would want to have answered; we also outlined the gains we think its adoption would offer for the processes of devising and reviewing of multi-location studies and clinical research protocols in general. Anyone who has tried publicly to suggest the development of a uniform, standardised *pro-forma* will have encountered the understandable reluctance with which individual RECs regard abandoning their own cherished and perhaps oft-modified version, on whose development dedicated members have spent much energy. This is indeed understandable, but it ought not to be allowed to obstruct the real benefits of adopting the best features of the best existing examples. Provided that a standardised *pro-forma* is sensibly and carefully geared towards getting these answers, then there is nothing of substance to be gained by digging in one's heels over a preferred form of words – and there is much to be lost.

12.2.2 Ineffectiveness of ethical review

In addition to the causes of frustration presented by the inefficiency of the system of ethical review of multi-location clinical research we discovered that researchers were concerned at the **ineffectiveness** of that review. Their concern seemed justified to the extent that the review system failed to provide them with the kind of guidance and support they expected from it. We further concluded that the system did not really provide the degree of protection properly owed to research subjects. These shortcomings arose in at least the following ways:

The variability of recommendations

The responses of local RECs to particular protocols was often extremely varied. Whilst differences in local conditions could properly account for some differences in recommendation, the nature of the disagreements went far beyond anything such differences could account for. It was clear that there was considerable variation in the criteria which the committees applied. Some demanded far more detailed information sheets than others; some were distracted by extraneous considerations – for example inter-professional tensions which made certain kinds of research difficult to process through ethical review. And demands for amendments to the protocols as such, reflecting these differences between committees, produced obvious difficulties in preserving the integrity and consistency of the protocols across all the areas where the study was to be pursued[10].

Lack of expertise on Local Research Ethics Committees

We received a number of complaints from researchers who conducted observational or analytic studies rather than clinical trials to the effect that in their experience most ethical review committees were well informed about and well equipped to assess only those protocols which approximated more or less to randomised controlled trials. These researchers claimed that a lack of the requisite expertise on some committees provoked unnecessary and ill-informed objections regarding, for instance, observational protocols, owing to the committees' unfamiliarity with the methodology of the protocols presented. Most committees, researchers believed, felt that 'hard science' like controlled trials was what clinical research was really about and had less regard for what was regarded as 'soft research'. Thus epidemiologists believed that many committees fell short of understanding the methodological character of protocols they submitted and, as a result, wrongly identified ethical problems in those protocols. Other researchers concerned with qualitative research shared the same feelings. Such suspicion has not abated in the period since our Report. Only very recently a working party of the Welsh National Board of Nursing and Midwifery, in a discussion paper about ethical review, complained of amendments requested by RECs simply because committee members were unfamiliar with the methodologies of nursing research[11].

It is true that even the different phases of pharmaceutical development present different challenges to an ethical review committee. Phase I research, which is usually not of a multi-location kind, involves the use of healthy volunteers and raises novel questions about the recruitment and reimbursement of subjects presenting ethical issues not presented by Phase II and III research (see section 6.3 above). This phase of pharmaceutical development also involves careful attention to pre-clinical research which local RECs have to consider on only relatively rare occasions (as indeed they rarely have to review Phase I research itself). When review is uninformed and lacks specialist experience and expertise, it obstructs the efficient and effective processing of research protocols.

The variability of practice of review committees

As we noted in section 8.4, some committees which we studied relied very heavily on chairman's action. One committee met simply to confirm or possibly review the chairman's action since the previous meeting, whilst another did all its reviewing by mail as the chairman thought necessary. In contrast some other committees demanded sufficient copies of full protocols to circulate to all their members, and others additionally demanded the presence of researchers to answer questions about the protocol. Whilst we warmly commend the practice of interviewing researchers as something which makes for thorough review, if every local REC demanded this on every occasion it would make the task of processing large multi-location protocols through the review process almost impossible under the present system. In sum, given the variation in RECs' practices, the coordinators of multi-location research found themselves trying to respond to such a range of different demands that it became nearly impossible to plan their way through the process of ethical review.

Relations between local and central review committees

Many multi-centre research protocols are initially reviewed by central committees, who are associated either with various professional sections of the clinical community or with formal research sponsors. These committees' approval is reported to the local RECs. We found that local reactions to this approval varied considerably. It was annoying to members of local committees to discover that the researcher had been told that, as central approval had been obtained, she could submit the research to the local committee for information if she so wished! Such suggestions are contrary to the Department of Health *Guidelines*, however authoritative the central committee might be[12]. Similarly some Hospital Trusts have set up ethical review committees and on occasion have falsely suggested that their approval does away with the need for approval by the local REC.

Local committees were rightly concerned that the review of each protocol be independent of both professional and managerial interests and that it be seen to be so. In the most extreme case we found that relations between one local REC and a certain central committee had so deteriorated that any protocol bearing the *imprimatur* of the central committee was turned down by the local committee on principle. Clearly such uncomfortable relations are ineffective, destructive and dangerous.

Quality control of ethical review

The variability in practice and performance of local RECs has really come to light most clearly in the multi-location context, when several of them are simultaneously considering and responding to the same protocol. As well as the problems this poses for multi-location research, it highlights the more general need for some kind of quality control in ethical review. A reform of the system of multi-location review offers an excellent opportunity for the introduction of quality assurance measures. However, it is important to recognise that quality assurance requires some sort of control mechanism. Two recent documents issued by the Department of Health attempt to describe, in formal terms, the standards which RECs should meet[13]. However helpful such documents might be in terms of informing RECs and their members, in themselves they offer no means of checking that the standards are actually being reached. For that, some means of monitoring and assessment is necessary. Reform of the system of multi-location review could involve a mechanism of notifying and comparing the different responses of different committees, at least so far as their review of the same protocols was concerned. Central advisory committees of the kind we shall describe below could play this rôle, but it's important not to confuse the idea of monitoring RECs' decisions with the quite separate idea of providing a means of appealing against them. (As things stand now, we don't see a plausible solution to the question of an appeals mechanism. We'll say more about this in section 12.4.2.)

12.3   Resolving the problems of multi-location review

I do wish the more suspicious of our G.P.s would stop feeling nervously
for their wallets every time I mention the word 'reform'.
(Rt. Hon. Kenneth Clarke, when Secretary of State for Health)

We have divided the various problems that came to light in the course of our research project into two groups, those concerning inefficiency and those concerning ineffectiveness. We concluded that the problems of inefficiency in the current system arose from its cumbersome nature, seen chiefly in the numbers of committees which have to be consulted and the wide variety of means which they employed to obtain the information they required from researchers. And we concluded that the problems of ineffectiveness of the current system arose from RECs' lack of specialised expertise on research methodologies, their inadequate liaison with central committees, the central committes' lack of perceived independence and, finally, local RECs' variability in practice and performance. Each of these major problems has to be faced.

In agreeing to make recommendations to the Department of Health on how the system could be reformed so as to resolve these problems, we found we had accepted a poisoned chalice. On one side there were vigorous advocates of a central national ethical review committee as the once-and-for-all solution to all problems, and on the other side were the equally vigorous and far more numerous defenders of RECs' autonomy and authority. It was clear that any solution would displease somebody for most of the time, and it soon became clear that any sensible compromise solution would displease everybody for at least some of the time. However, since we thought that elements of both central review and local scrutiny were important, some such compromise was called for as a means to streamlining the system whilst preserving the quality of review. The compromise we recommended is outlined below; whilst we set no particular store on the precise form of the package as a whole, the elements making it up still seem to us to be necessary elements in any acceptable reform. Before outlining the recommendations made in that research project and before considering other possible combinations of its elements, we need to recognise the inevitable tension between the two goals of achieving efficiency on the one hand and effectiveness on the other.

12.3.1 Balancing efficiency and effectiveness

We are taking it as read that there can be no ethical justification for unnecessary delays in the ethical review of clinical research; the necessity of any justified delay would have to consist in meeting some ethically important requirement, for instance the obtaining of vital additional information. But by the same token there can be no ethical justification for ineffective review. Ineffective review could be more dangerous than no review at all: an ill-grounded approval might encourage researchers to proceed uncritically with research projects which, had they not received such approval, they might have subjected to self-regulation of a more rigorous kind. Now we have seen that efficiency and effectiveness can come into conflict; a clear case arises under the present system if every local REC insisted on interviewing the coordinating researcher of a large multi-location project. To preserve the present system and make it workable in this respect, it would seem that we should have to require RECs to settle for less than the best practice.

Whilst it is tempting to pursue the gains of increased efficiency first and foremost, given the pressures from researchers and sponsors of research, this would be a serious mistake. The most efficient system of ethical review might turn out to be an extremely shabby affair which seriously failed to achieve the main objective of ethical review, viz. the protection of the safety and interests of research subjects. Whilst delays in research involve penalties to the interests of other vulnerable parties, particularly future patients, we have proceeded throughout this book on the basis that the REC's primary concern is with the protection of the research subject. This means that, where they conflict, effectiveness of review **must** come before efficiency. The Declaration of Helsinki points out unambiguously that in no circumstances should these priorities be reversed:

> The purpose of Biomedical research involving human subjects must be to improve diagnostic, therapeutic and prophylactic procedures and the understanding of the aetiology and pathogenesis of disease...Every biomedical research project involving human subjects should be preceded by careful assessment of predictable risks in comparison with forseeable benefits to the subject and to others. **Concern for the interests of the subject must always prevail over the interest of science and society.**[14]

Thus if the price of proper protection of research subjects' interests is a system in which some delays are inevitable, then provided they are kept to a reasonable minimum those delays are ethically justified.

12.3.2   The elements of a solution

Our recommendations for reforming the system of multi-location ethical review contained few new elements. We modified and developed already-existing features of the review system, chiefly including the use of **lead committees** (such as were proposed in the Department of Health's *Guidelines*[15]) and the employment of **advisory committees** (a role already played by various central committees such as the Ethics Committees of the Royal College of General Practitioners and the Public Health Laboratory Service, in-house committees of pharmaceutical houses and *ad hoc* ethical review committees of sponsors of clinical research such as the Medical Research Council). These features we combined with a modified rôle for local RECs specifically in multi-location review; their rôle in the review of other research was unchanged and unaffected.

However, whilst none of these elements was new, in considering and recommending precise rôles for these bodies we drew on an important distinction that had really not been fully appreciated or emphasised in previous attention to the problems of multi-location review. This is the distinction – set out above in section 11.5 – between on the one hand the general conception and form of a particular piece of research, and on the other hand the special features and context of applying that piece of research locally. It is one thing to approve the scientific and ethical content of a protocol in the abstract (what we have called the 'protocol as such'); it is quite another to know when it is to be entrusted to particular researchers, working in particular clinical facilities, with a particular patient population. On the basis of this distinction we identified the two distinct **stages** of ethical review as being in a sense 'physically' separable in the particular context of multi-location review. The two stages could constitute distinct rôles for distinct bodies.

Once the rôle of the different bodies is spelled out then the next questions concern who they should be and how many of them will be needed. There are various permutations of number and identity which more or less address different problems identified in the system. In this chapter we will not be concerned to recommend any particular combination so much as to note the range of possibilities, and to point out both the expected benefits and the likely price of each possibility.

Lead committees

The UK Department of Health's revised *Guidelines*, published in 1991, recognised that there were problems in processing multi-centre research through ethical review and made a proposal for the resolution of these problems. The solution reads as follows:

> Each LREC is free to arrive at its own decision when considering a proposal which is planned to take place in more than one area. It would, however, obviously be sensible – in the interests of eliminating unnecessary delay and of ensuring that similar criteria are used to consider a proposal – that committees should arrive at a voluntary arrangement under which one LREC is nominated to consider the issue on behalf of them all. Health authorities should positively encourage networks for neighbouring LRECs so that such co-operation is more easily achieved.[16]

Here we find the concept of a lead committee. Such a committee would consider a given research protocol on behalf of a number of other committees and its approval or disapproval would by implication be binding on those other committees. (Although this is not stated in the *Guidelines*, the 'one-for-all' arrangement falls apart if the other RECs take it upon themselves to review the decision of the nominated committee; the only alternative is that they simply accept it and are bound by it.) Thus taking a lead would be more rigorous than setting an example. It would be the beginning and the end of the process of ethical review for that particular research project for all the committees in question – for both the stages of review which we distinguished above. In effect this means that there is no real review of the local **implementation** of the proposed research, except at most in the area local to the nominated committee. Thereafter, if any new centre or location under the jurisdiction of those committees were to be the venue for the execution of an arm of that research project, then no further approval would need to be sought from the local committee of that area and such a committee would have no power to amend the protocol as such, nor – so far as the *Guidelines* describe it – to challenge the suitability of local implementation.

Advisory committees

At present local RECs in the United Kingdom may benefit from the advice of central committees such as those mentioned above. That advice is almost always limited to the information that such and such a central committee has approved the study. Occasionally such central advice purports to carry the authority of decisions of lead committees but such claims are false: no lead committees have yet been authorised to act as such. Nevertheless, in our research we discovered that large numbers of members of local RECs were impressed in various ways by such minimal advice.[17] Almost a quarter of our respondents (22.8%) said that they felt under pressure to approve multi-centre trials which had already been passed by another committee. A very small number (2.1%) felt that a central committee's decision was decisive whilst a further 60.7% felt that it was very important; 6% of respondents strongly agreed and 37.3% agreed with the idea that central committees were better qualified than LRECs. A small proportion (2.3%) believed that LREC review of such protocols was an unnecessary obstacle to research whilst a larger group (6.1%) thought it was a wasteful duplication. When asked to consider the proposition that local RECs should **not** have the power to veto centrally approved protocols, 3.6% of our respondents strongly agreed and a further 12.8% agreed that they should not have such power – almost one in six REC members. When asked to consider the proposition that the review of multi-centre trials should never be taken out of the hands of local RECs 3.0% strongly disagreed and a further 19.5% disagreed with the view.

Clearly, then, many REC members see a place for a central advisory body in the review process despite their generally fierce defence of local independence and autonomy.

12.3.3 Our initial recommendations

The extent of local REC involvement

We regard each of the two stages of ethical review, distinguished above in section 11.5, as absolutely essential. Moreover, only a local body can possibly assess the circumstances on its own 'patch'. Given the proper rôle, expertise and experience of local RECs in reviewing the implementation of all the other, non-multi-location research which falls within their remit, they are the obvious bodies to carry this responsibility in multi-location research as well. These considerations alone, independently of RECs' own views on their independence and autonomy, point to an inviolable rôle for them in reviewing at least the implementation of research.

But need they be involved in more than this, specifically in the first stage of ethical review? We recognised that the problems of the current system are inextricably tied to local RECs being fully involved in both elements of the review process; reforming the current system seems to demand that this involvement be restricted. Obviously we must ask whether anything vital would be lost if their involvement were substantially restricted to reviewing local implementation only. One thing would certainly be lost – the very wide pool of peer review which is presently able to suggest modifications to a protocol would shrink dramatically and, to paraphrase what we said earlier on, if peer review is a good thing then dramatically less of it looks like a big step backwards. On the face of it this is a substantial objection. Its force, however, must be tested against two considerations. First, it must be tested against how often in practice the broad pool of local REC reviewers make genuine improvements to the general design of a protocol. It's not easy to demonstrate that this happens at all often, even though REC members might like to believe it to be a routine occurrence. Second, it must be tested against the effectiveness of whatever is put in place of wholesale REC involvement. Clearly then the objection can't be used to oppose the **principle** of reform; it does, however, remind us that a benchmark for any more efficient system is that it be at least as effective as the current pool of peer review. That is a goal we have kept in our sights throughout our recommendations.

The number and identity of advisory committees

In response to researchers' concerns that local RECs often lacked expertise across the range of research methodologies, the need for RECs to be advised on those methodologies by properly qualified bodies – central advisory committees – seemed clear enough. The main questions to be answered were how many such committees were required and what their composition should be.

We looked at the conventional proposal to set up a National Ethics Committee to review all multi-location clinical research protocols. This would have a membership of acknowledged experts in clinical research who would serve in an independent capacity insofar as they would not represent any particular interest group in medicine, nursing or any other clinical field. To the extent that local RECs recognised their expertise and their independence from particular sectional interests, then the advice which they offered could make a positive contribution to the performance of ethical review at the local level. But the advice which RECs need should be more than just an announcement of approval by another committee. It should consist in a precise and detailed summary of the major issues considered by the reviewing committee, giving its reasons for approving or amending the protocol which is eventually presented for consideration to the local REC. In this way an advisory body could play an important educative role in the system of ethical review, helping not only in the local review of multi-centre protocols but also in the review of all other protocols considered by local committees. The input of such advice would also go a long way to resolving the doubts about requisite expertise in ethical review in the minds of researchers.

We concluded that advice of this kind would indeed require a central body to provide it, since the required range of expertise would be unlikely to be available to any local committee or even regional committee. However, we were also persuaded that no one committee of manageable size could cope with either the volume of business or the diversity of research categories represented in multi-location research activity nationally. We therefore suggested that specialised expert committees be set up for three groupings of research:

(a) Phase III pharmaceutical trials and non-pharmaceutical trials of similar design – e.g. research into the use of new surgical techniques in randomised controlled trials;

(b) Phase IV pharmaceutical trials including post-marketing surveillance (such as is described in Section 4 of Appendix A of the Department of Health *Guidelines* on LRECs);

(c) epidemiological and behavioural research[18].

The number and identity of lead committees

The suggestion that lead committees be employed at all in ethical review provokes hostile reactions from large sections of the membership of local RECs, as we learned very quickly after presenting our recommendations at the Royal College of Physicians. However, we see no realistic alternative to using them if the process of review of multi-centre research is to be streamlined. And we think that if the lead committees were properly selected then resistance from local RECs would decline. At the same time, if the selection were not made carefully then introducing lead committees would be counterproductive. This is because any lack of confidence which RECs felt towards the lead committees would incline them to resist protocols which those committees had approved. If local implementation of research is to remain a matter for review by the local Committee – as we are convinced it should – then the local Committee has always got the option of advising its local Health Authority against permitting the research locally. This gives it an effective veto over research, even if it lost the power to amend the protocol as such. We will return to this consideration shortly.

It was our proposal that there be a limited number of lead committees, all of which would have to agree on a recommendation to approve any research before that research could begin. We suggested that the best way to win the confidence of local committees would be for them to play a part in the working of the lead committees. This would be made possible by setting up about twelve regional committees throughout the United Kingdom, each representing about twelve local committees and drawing its members from those local committees. If all twelve considered multi-location protocols then every area of the country would be represented in the approval mechanism and it would be open to the coordinators of any such project to carry out the research anywhere it wished to, provided the local REC supported its implementation. We have already pointed out that there are relatively few country-wide research projects; where fewer regions were affected then correspondingly fewer regional committees would need to be consulted. In our experience of reviewing multi-location research this would typically reduce the number of lead committees involved to five or fewer.

The role of lead committees has to be coordinated with the responsibilities of the local RECs. We have already discussed in some detail those responsibilities that only local committees can properly acquit (sections 11.5 and 12.3.2). Local RECs should therefore review the local implementation of research – and approve or refuse it as appropriate – according to strictly limited criteria. They would not have the power to amend the protocol as such but might be given limited powers to amend information sheets and consent forms to allow for special local circumstances, such as the language difficulties of some sections of the pool of potential research subjects.

We rejected the Department of Health *Guidelines*' suggestion that a single selected local REC should play the role of lead committee. We did so for a number of reasons apart from our conviction that the quality of overall review would be improved by involving several such committees rather than a single committee, given that no one committee could be expected to be all-knowing. Our most important reason was that from the evidence we collected from the wide range of committees we examined we realised that no single local committee would command the necessary respect of all the rest – and without the confidence of the RECs at the stage of reviewing implementation, the system simply cannot work. When we sought responses from individual committees to the ideas underlying our recommendations, we found there was one feature which they all had in common: each committee was certain that it performed the task of ethical review in the best manner. In addition we noted that almost 60% of members who responded to our questionnaire rejected the Department of Health's *Guidelines* suggestion; 49.2% disagreed and a further 9.8% strongly disagreed with the view that multi-location ethical review would be best handled by the use of local RECs as lead committees.

Variations on the *Guidelines* suggestion might improve its viability, though these were defined too late to be included in our survey. One variation is to put all the RECs in a particular region on a rota so that each acts as the lead committee in its turn. Whilst appearing even-handed, this approach guarantees that from time to time all multi-location review in that region is handled by the REC least competent to do it. A more promising variation would distribute responsibility for multi-location review amongst several RECs in each region, on a similar basis to the classification of the central advisory committees, defining the clinical or methodological field of a piece of research and putting review in the hands of the REC most experienced in that field. But neither of these variations seems to us to be as acceptable or as effective as regional, 'composite' committees whose members were drawn from the RECs they represented.

The three-tier solution

Our recommendation in 1992 was that the most effective ethical review of a given protocol would be achieved by using an appropriate central advisory committee to handle the application and all correspondence with the proposer of the research, and to make a general scientific and ethical review of the protocol on an advisory basis. When satisfied that ultimate approval would be appropriate, the advisory comittee would distribute the protocol to the requisite number of regional lead committees. Any disagreements at this level would be reported back to the central committee which would ask the researcher to amend the protocol accordingly. Once agreement had been reached between the lead committees then any researcher would be free to apply to begin the research in his or her area through the local committee, which would check on local criteria.

(Initially we thought that all the lead committees' approval should be necessary for the protocol to proceed further. This might be too stringent a requirement. But there is an important rôle for dissenting voices in a majority approval at this stage. The reasons for any lead committee's unhappiness could be notified to the others, giving them the opportunity to reconsider their approval if they thought it appropriate – but not requiring them to do so.)

Amongst the responses to the proposal three criticisms were made which we think can be answered. The first was that the system would be too bureaucratic. It is true that a secretariat would have to be set up to service the central committees and liaise with researchers and committees. This would, however, replace what is generally agreed in the research world to be a chaotic mish-mash of communications between researchers and very large numbers of convenors of local RECs, each of whom might have his or her own views of what is reasonable in the way of response times and the documentary forms of information required. To put it bluntly, it is partly the **lack** of a proper bureaucratic machinery which makes the processing of multi-centre protocols through ethical review such a headache for researchers. Thus we make no apology for recommending a more bureacratic system.   Whether the precise one which we recommended is too bureaucratic depends on how thorough are the demands that people should make regarding the quality of ethical review, and on what alternative reforms could be produced to bring about both quality and speed at the same time.

Another criticism was that the recommendations were too time-consuming.   We found this somewhat puzzling, given the interminable delays endemic in the current system.   We tried to set out a timetable for the processing of the toughest case – the nationwide research protocol – through the system as reformed according to our recommendations.   We predicted, perhaps a little optimistically, that an application could be turned around in three months.   We still think that this is not far short of the mark.   We are, after all, simply suggesting the passage of each protocol through a maximum of thirteen committees, all but one of which would consider it simultaneously (and this with the aid of a central secretariat) before going directly to the local RECs for a much more restricted review within the criteria for local implementation.   For most multi-centre trials the numbers would be much smaller.

Finally, it was complained that the three-tier system was excessive.   Presumably this criticism was aimed at the **number** of committees required to consider each protocol.   When compared with the current system – where in a nationwide project some 150-plus committees are expected to review each protocol in full – the proposed scheme seems modest in the demands it makes.   Even in much more limited (and much more typical) multi-location research, the protocol as such will be reviewed by only one lead committee per region where it is proposed the research should actually be carried out.   In most instances this too represents a substantial saving.   Of course our scheme is not as 'slim' as schemes which eradicated the advisory tier, nor as schemes which reduced the number of lead committees to one.   But in making these restricted demands we have to balance efficiency against the effectiveness of the review which is achieved.

Thus, whilst we accept that our recommended three-tier system is not the only possible solution to the problems of the review of multi-location research, alternative reforms which do away with any of the elements in our own scheme must be scrutinised to see whether in the process they lose anything of importance.   In the Annexe to this chapter (pp. 195-6) we will set out various possible combinations of the elements discussed above and compare in a tabular form the advantages and disadvantages of adopting each of them.   We shall not review the possibility of single-tier arrangements using either central, regional or local lead committees; these cut out the local review of research **implementation** altogether and make it impossible to protect research subjects properly from such hazards as under-qualified researchers, over-worked researchers, inadequate research facilities, specific demographic and population concerns, over-exposed cohorts of patients and so on. We think such protections are simply non-negotiable in any ethical review worthy of the name, and reforms which did away with these protections would be totally unacceptable. We will, however, set out other possible two- and three-tier combinations, and these must be judged sensitively in terms of how securely they can gain efficiency without weakening the protection of the research subject.

12.4 Remaining difficulties in multi-location review

Streets flooded. Please advise.
(Robert Benchley, in a telegram from Venice.)

There are two further difficulties which have to be addressed in any reform of the system of multi-location ethical review. These difficulties crop up in the review of all clinical research protocols, but they are particularly highlighted in the context of multi-location review. Reforming the multi-location arrangements offers valuable spin-off gains for the more general review of clinical protocols.

12.4.1 Financing ethical review

If ethical review is as serious a matter as everyone says it is, then it deserves proper financing. In the United Kingdom this important service has, until now, been provided on a shoe-string budget. We acknowledged in section 8.7 above the problems of the merely honorary status of REC members. Reforming the multi-location context encourages the search for standardised and properly regulated solutions to common problems. There could, for instance, be a strict tariff of payments to REC members, subject to guidelines from the appropriate national body (in the U.K. it would be the Department of Health) in order to be seen to guarantee the probity of ethical review. There is actually a successful precedent for a **professional** committee performing the task of ethical review, and it illustrates one approach to the problem of funding the review process. The Food and Drug Administration in the United States contracts out ethical review to at least one commercial body of this sort[19]. The committeee is financed by the direct billing of the sponsor – there being a set levy for the process of ethical review of protocols. The members of that committee are paid a fee for each protocol they examine and the full-time chairman's salary and administration expenses of the committee are also covered by the levy. Such a measure demands very strict oversight and control by the employing agency, which itself must have no vested interest in the outcome of the committee's deliberations.

Now the rôle of the above committee is limited to the review of multi-centre clinical trials which have been referred to the FDA as part of the process of satisfying the conditions for licensing new medicines. (Of course, where any committee of this sort is used for reviewing multi-centre protocols as a 'lead committee', it incurs all the drawbacks of single-committee review which we noted earlier.) The sponsoring organisations are the pharmaceutical houses which are pleased to pay the levy in order to enjoy the benefits of accelerated review and minimal delay in the clinical development time of their medicines. In the United Kingdom Research Ethics Committees have a much wider brief and whilst they do consider protocols from this source they also consider large numbers of protocols from individual researchers and small clinical and academic departments. The trouble with imposing a general levy for ethical review is that it could on the one hand discourage research or, on the other hand, tempt researchers struggling on tight budgets to avoid the ethical review process altogether. Either of these consequences would be highly undesirable and would threaten the interests of both research subjects and future patients. The obvious alternative, which is to charge differential levies, runs up against the problem of deciding who is capable of paying what; and it would obviously discriminate against pharmaceutical companies, research charities and government sponsors. (On the other hand, it seems obvious that even an 'unfair' system of this kind is still substantially in the interests of the pharmaceutical industry, given the significant economic gains it could expect from efficiency reforms.)

It is a fact that, even without payments for the time and services of individual members of RECs, the system of ethical review in the United Kingdom is already grossly underfinanced. District Health Authorities have inadequate allowances to afford proper servicing of their RECs in the form of convenors' time, secretarial facilities, data collection and analysis and so on. So a considerable injection of funds is needed in any case. Raising funds at the level of the local REC would vastly increase the burdens of an already overworked administration. It therefore seems to us that central government funding should be provided, preferably out of the general provision for Research & Development budgets. Perhaps research sponsors in the form of organisations of pharmaceutical companies and research charities could be encouraged to pay one-off sums annually into such centrally administered funds in return for considerable savings on effective patent time and research costs. This way of channelling the financial support of interested parties would also be seen to be free of any appearance of buying approval from specific committees and it would preserve the independence of the ethical review procedure.

12.4.2   Quality assurance of ethical review and appeal procedures

Providing quality assurance

The Department of Health has taken some steps in the United Kingdom to address the problem of quality assurance in ethical review, publishing documents in 1995 on RECs' goals, competencies and standard operating procedures in an effort to produce a more uniform and acceptable performance from local committees. However, advisory documents, as we noted, entail no monitoring or control of standards; in practice they leave RECs free to proceed however they wish.

This difficulty of quality assurance of ethical review is not peculiar to the United Kingdom. For example, in the course of our research for the Department of Health we examined some efforts to address precisely the same issue in the United States. There the Office of Protection from Research Risks (OPRR) tries to keep track of the ethical review procedures concerning those clinical research protocols sponsored by the National Institutes of Health. It does so by comparing the performance of different committees (known there as Institutional Review Boards) in terms of the approvals, disapprovals or requests for amendment which they issue. If any given committee's performance appears out of step with the general pattern then its decisions are carefully scrutinised; if the OPRR feels that the Committee is in need of advice or help in improving its performance it attempts to provide the assistance required. This is only the beginning of a quality assurance mechanism but the OPRR is eager to improve on it.

The United States' Food and Drug Administration also has some statutory backing in that satisfactory ethical review is a legal requirement in the licensing process of new medicines in the United States. The Administration therefore has legally to provide an inspectorate to monitor the performance of Institutional Review Boards. Inspectors are authorised to carry out spot-checks on committees and to examine all the paperwork relating to the review procedure.   The problem with this kind of quality assurance mechanism is that it is both very expensive, in that a large number of personnel have to be appointed to carry out inspections, and of only limited effectiveness as inspection tends to be bureaucratic and superficial.   A thorough inspection would need staff who were highly expert in evaluating the quality of discussion in review meetings and in research methodology and who would sit through the deliberations of IRBs.   This would be an vastly expensive scheme to set up, if indeed it were possible to set it up at all.

The reform of the procedure for reviewing multi-location clinical research protocols in the United Kingdom offers the opportunity to introduce a quality assurance mechanism which would develop the promising model of the OPRR.   The problem with that model as it is employed in the United States is that a significant number of poor performances have to occur before the detection system is even alerted to the possibility of a problem: in order to work, the system needs first to fail!   On the basis that prevention is better than cure we propose that, given the use of a central ethical review committee in an advisory role, that committee play a monitoring role of the performance of local RECs. This could be done fairly easily by such a committee's periodically processing test protocols (either real or invented) through all local RECs and comparing the results.   Obvious flaws or anomalies in review practice should thus come to light and the central committee could take remedial action by alerting the committees in question to their shortcomings, and perhaps by requiring them to undergo some relevant training to correct the problems.   This would be a relatively cheap but nonetheless effective way of providing quality assurance in the system of ethical review;   as we noted in section 8.8, training facilities which could be used by such committees are available in the United Kingdom now.

The question of an appeals procedure

Given that lead committees will have the power to refuse approval for given protocols, and given also that they might disagree amongst themselves on their recommendations, the question arises as to whether an appeals procedure should be set up.   If this means using a central committee as a 'court' of appeal, then we are against the idea.   Take, to begin with, the lead committees' review of the protocols as such.   If these committees are set up to be properly competent to decide whether protocols are acceptable in principle, there is no reason to think that a central committee would enjoy any greater authority. If lead committees disagree over any particular protocol, then researchers could ask those lead committees which withheld approval to reconsider their decision in the light of the contrary decisions of other committees. The dissenting lead committee should do this in good faith, but if not persuaded to change their decision then they should stand by it.

As regards the local review of implementation of research, no central committee could be better placed than the local committee to decide whether the criteria for local implementation of a research protocol are satisfied. To grant a distant body power to overrule a local decision would undermine the principle of responsibility for the execution of local research which devolves on the local REC.

Note on the Annexe

The systems tabled on pages 195-6 have been proposed by various contributors to the general discussion on the best means to multi-location review. Their advantages and disadvantages are listed here in a summary form as we envisage them; the items express substantive points which we discussed in the text. Although they appear as items in a list, they are not all of equal weight, and whilst a given advantage or disadvantage may appear in more than one system of review it cannot be assumed that it would have equal force, or be experienced to the same extent, in each system. This table is simply a guide to what we think could be expected under any of the systems.

Notes

1   Friedman, L.M., Furberg, C.D. and DeMets, D.L., *Fundamentals of Clinical Trials*, Boston: John Wright/PSG Inc. (1981), Table 7.3, p. 77.

2   *ibid.*

3   Pelerin, M. and Hall, S., 'Ethics and multi-centre research projects', correspondence, *British Medical Journal*, 304 (1992), p. 1696.

4   See Walker, S., Girling, L. and Prentice, R., 'Innovation and the availability of medicines', *The Pharmaceutical Journal*, 234 (1985), pp. 264-6.

5   Walker, S.R. and Parrish, A.J., 'Innovation and new drug development', in Walker, B.C. and Walker, S.R., (eds), *Trends and Changes in Drug Research and Development*, London: Kluwer Academic Publishers (1988), pp. 19, 22.

6   We are grateful to the Centre for Medicines Research for these and the following data.

7   For this figure see Grabowski, H.G. and Vernon, J.M. *The Regulation of Pharmaceuticals: Balancing the Benefits and Risks*, Washington D.C. & London: American Enterprise Institute (1983).

8   Some proposals for such *pro-forma* documents have been made recently.   For example see Doyal,L., 'Towards a standard application form for LRECs', *Bulletin of Medical Ethics*, 101 (1994), pp. 15-28.

9   Pleas for a standardised *pro-forma* application form continue to be made. See for instance Robbins, G., 'Ethics committees', *The Lancet*, 345 (1995), p. 653.

10   This continues to be lamented: see for instance Hotopf, M., Wessely and S., Noah, N., 'Are ethical committees reliable?', *Journal of the Royal Society of Medicine*, 88 (1995), pp. 31-3.

11   Welsh Nursing and Midwifery Committee, *Multi-centre Research Issues Paper*, Cardiff: Welsh National Board of Nursing and Midwifery (1995), p.3.

12   The Department of Health's *Guidelines* state categorically that 'An LREC must be **consulted** about any research proposal involving ... NHS patients [or]... access to the records of past or present NHS patients...' *inter alia* (paragraph 1.3, our emphasis).

13   National Health Service Training Division, *Standards for Local Research Ethics Committees*, London: Department of Health (1994);   Bendall, C., *Standard Operating Procedures for Local Research Ethics Committees*, London: McKenna & Co. (1994).

14   World Medical Association Declaration of Helsinki: *Recommendations Guiding Medical Doctors in Biomedical Research Involving Human Subjects*, adopted by the 18th World Medical Assembly, Helsinki, Finland, 1964, and revised by the 29th World Medical Assembly, Tokyo, Japan, 1975; Introduction and I:5. (The emphasis in the extract is ours.)

15   Department of Health, *Local Research Ethics Committees*, para. 2.18.

16   *ibid.*

17   The research questionnaire on multi-centre review was sent out to all local RECs in England. It enjoyed a response from 75% of those committees and individual responses from 70% of members of those committees.

18   These are the groupings recommended in our Report; the rationale for the third grouping was more one of combined volume than of considerations of methodology, and of course it could be criticised on that account.

19   The Essex Institutional Review Board, New Jersey, U.S.A., Chairman, W.Waggoner.

Annexe to Chapter Twelve: various proposals for systems of multilocation review

System	Tiers	Advantages	Disadvantages
Central lead committee, limited local review	two	- guarantees expert review - greatly reduces complexity and delay - local consideration of implementation - offers gains in efficiency - avoids costs of regional committees	- minimal local involvement risks RECs' local veto - single lead committee reduces effectiveness - additional expense of convening central committee - -may not expedite research in practice
Local lead committee, limited local review	two	- greatly reduces complexity and delay - avoids costs of central or regional committees - local consideration of implementation - offers gains in efficiency	- minimal local involvement risks RECs' local veto - single lead committee reduces effectiveness - no acknowledged authority in protocol review - loses educative benefits of central advisory committee - may greatly sacrifice effectiveness for efficiency - may not expedite research in practice
Central advisory committee, full local review	two	- guarantees expert review - ensures full cooperation of local RECs - offers educative support to local RECs - full review of protocols and of implementation - avoids costs of regional committees - gains in effectiveness	- worse delays even than present system - adds to frustration of researchers and sponsors - additional expense of convening central committee - sacrifices efficiency for marginal extra effectiveness - may hinder research in practice
Regional advisory committee, full local review	two	- ensures full cooperation of local RECs - offers educative support to local RECs - avoids costs of central committee(s)	- no acknowledged authority in advice on protocols - additional expense of regional committees - worse delays than present system - adds to frustration of researchers and sponsors - sacrifices efficiency for marginal gain in effectiveness

(continued)

Annexe to Chapter Twelve (continued)

System	Tiers	Advantages	Disadvantages
Regional lead committee, limited local review	two	- encourages cooperation of RECs - reduces complexity and delay - avoids cost of central committees - local consideration of implementation	- no acknowledged authority in advice on protocols - additional expense of regional committees - single lead committee reduces effectiveness - may sacrifice effectiveness for greater efficiency
Central advisory, regional lead committee/s, plus limited local review	three	- provides expert review - educative input for RECs - effective review if several lead committees used - simplifies administration of review, reduces delay - local review of implementation - reassures RECs - offers increased efficiency and effectiveness	- reduces effectiveness if single lead committee used - additional expense of central committee(s) - additional expense of regional committee(s) - appearance of complexity - may considerably increase cost of review process
Central advisory, local lead committee/s, plus limited local review	three	- expert advisory input - educative input for RECs - effective review if several lead committees used - simplifies administration of review, reduces delay - local review of implementation - avoids cost of regional committees - offers increased efficiency (and effectiveness?)	- reduces effectiveness if single lead committee used - additional expense of central committee - loss of REC cooperation - problems of identifying suitable local lead committee - appearance of complexity - may not expedite research in practice
Regional advisory, local lead committee/s, plus limited local review	three	- some educative support - effective review if several lead committees used - simplifies administration of review, reduces delay - local review of implementation - avoids cost of central committees - offers increased efficiency (and effectiveness?)	- no acknowledged authority in advice on protocols - reduces effectiveness if single lead committee used - additional expense of regional committee(s) - loss of REC co-operation - problems of identifying suitable local lead committee - may not expedite research in practice

Chapter Thirteen

The future of ethical review

In this book we have been concerned first with the moral force of the requirement for ethical review of clinical research and second with the principles and practices that constitute good ethical review. We shall conclude by looking ahead to how the practice of ethical review and the rôle of RECs might develop or be extended, specifically in the United Kingdom context where the current practices of ethical review are both more recent and more narrowly restricted than in the United States. Throughout this chapter we are engaged in a discussion that is largely speculative. We will try to identify the considerations and arguments that are relevant to looking ahead in an informed way, and wherever possible we will look at existing precedents for the sorts of developments that we are envisaging. Even if none of these developments actually came about, the considerations and arguments relevant to them will remain relevant to present REC practice, and they spring out of the principles and practices that have occupied us until now.

13.1   Statutory ethical review of clinical research?

Let's find out what everyone is doing, and then stop everyone from doing it.
(A.P. Herbert)

In Chapter Ten we began our reflections on ethical review and the law by noting the absence of any statutory requirement for ethical review of research in Britain. Of those changes that could realistically be imagined, the biggest single change in the public profile of ethical review in the UK would be its acquiring the force of a legal duty. Quite how much difference this would make in practice is another matter, but in all likelihood its visibility amongst patients and research subjects would for the first time be guaranteed – particularly in an age where both self-conscious consumer expectations and the somewhat prodigal Charters which nowadays fuel those expectations can be found even in the domain of health care provision.   Presently, information about the processes of ethical review may be obscure, buried in appendices to consent forms or even absent altogether from the information given to prospective and actual research subjects. Of course it is a moot point whether those who are sick and vulnerable are more interested in the machinery guaranteeing their lawful expectations than they are in the care and comfort aimed at promoting their physical recovery.   What is much clearer is the importance of signalling to the international medical research industry that ethical review is a serious requirement and that the bodies to whom the process is entrusted mean business.   So it is not surprising that (as we noted in section 10.1) a prominent argument in favour of a statutory requirement for ethical review concerns the 'symbolic' or 'declaratory' rôle of the law.   This argument readily leads to another, namely that the international character of modern medical research should be matched by a uniformity and consistency across different nation-states and different legal jurisdictions.   Whilst even until recently it might privately have suited some within the industrial research community to find that in the least-regulated countries the research subject populations enjoy virtually no domestic protection whatever, today the research community as a whole knows full well that to export its products to the lucrative United States market it must satisfy the requirements of the U.S. Food and Drug Administration, which include specifications of the ethical review processes to be complied with regardless of the country in which the research was conducted.   The European Union is in the process of putting in place Directives which are uniformly binding on the E.U. member states in the matter of formally requiring ethical review processes[1]. Legislative untidiness or patchiness across different jurisdictions will in the long run be countered by political drives for uniformity or the simple practicalities of an entrance ticket to the world's richest therapeutic market.   So why not simply formalise the position and set in place harmonised statutory requirements for the highest common standards of ethical review in all the relevant countries?

Clearly, part of any argument against the statutory imposition of ethical review might be an appeal to these very practicalities: what's the point of legislation when any intelligent, self-interested attention to the profit motive will lead to the same result?   The 'razor' traditionally wielded by William of Occam to trim away the surplus fat of schoolmen's logic is just as relevant, and just as effective, in matters of the law: don't invent laws to compel the inevitable (or, in a more contemporary argot, 'If it ain't broke don't fix it').   A related, and at first sight more impressive, contention is that rules and more especially laws carry the danger of subduing the **moral** character of the concern which underlies voluntary arrangements or self-regulation. On inspection, however, it is not clear whether self-regulation of the kind to be found in research practices within, for instance, the National Health Service, or the procedural requirements for establishing RECs in the British public health care sector, are really spontaneous institutional expressions of moral concern rather than prudent administrative responses to the emergence of consumerism and the rise in health-related litigation. But again, noting this litigation invites a further objection to the claimed necessity of putting ethical review on a statutory footing: all the **legal** as well as the administrative protections which research subjects might need are already in place, in the laws concerning negligence, battery, assault, manslaughter and murder. If there are gaps in the protections offered by the relevant laws, those gaps need to be identified and shown to be capable of being closed by making ethical review statutory. And this seems most unlikely, unless new statutes created a new criminal offence of 'undertaking research in the absence of ethical approval' such that a conviction rendered the culprit (or her employing authority) liable for compensation to any injured party.

Part of the case for introducing new statutory controls must rest on being able to give a convincing account of the practical machinery necessary for its implementation: legal obligations must be ones that can reasonably be carried out. The simplest way of doing this is just to take the existing apparatus of ethical review and put it on a statutory footing; in this way a new law would be almost entirely formal, requiring the **fact** of ethical review rather than any particular pattern or method of it. This means, of course, formalising both the strengths and the weaknesses of the present system, unless at the same time steps are taken to make the system more effective (and such steps will cost money). We have spent much time in this book considering what goes into an effective standard of ethical discussion, in terms of what REC members ought to take into account when they prepare for and engage in the Committee's deliberations. The law is not likely to go into these matters (for instance, requiring and specifying training for REC members). If new legal specifications concerned themselves at all with the practicalities of the system of ethical review, they would more realistically be confined to the mechanics of administering the application procedures, perhaps with the maximum geographical spread or extent of an REC's remit, with the frequency of meetings or maximum workloads, with certain exemptions (such as research which is to be reviewed elsewhere, a matter we will touch on shortly), and with the formal requirements for publication of Annual Reports. Furthermore, it is likely that legal specifications would be couched in very general terms, requiring 'sufficient' or 'appropriate' coverage and workloads, and leaving it within the responsibility of a designated authority to fulfil the formal requirement of making sure that such a review 'service' were provided. None of this in itself offers any guarantee that ethical review will be taken more seriously than at present, leaving us with the symbolic value of such a law as being its most likely concrete benefit.

When thinking about the pros and cons of a hypothetical situation it is often very useful to look for a sufficiently close precedent and, if one can be found, to study it and consider whether conclusions can be drawn from it. Two precedents which suggest themselves are, first, actual statutory ethical review in a comparable country and, second, other comparable statutory measures in the United Kingdom.

The great difficulty with comparable countries lies in actually finding them. In Chapter One we considered the example of statutory ethical review found in the United States, but in contrast with the United Kingdom the U.S. is a geographically huge country with a correspondingly distinctive apparatus of Federal law and regulation and their institutional mechanisms; it also has a tradition which accepts and respects the idea of litigation as an individual's bulwark against the power of professionals. Denmark's statutory grounding of ethical review lies at the other end of the scale, with a relatively small population and a much smaller absolute degree of research activity to be controlled. It is not clear what difference has been made in practice by moving from an informally regulated to a statutory system[2]. France's longer established system of statutory ethical review reflects its greater administrative and legislative centralisation and its political tradition of intervention; and so on. Neither historical nor prospective randomised controls are easily obtained when it comes to distributing trial variables among nation-states; faced with this the scientific historian might settle for the more modest 'own control' approach of looking at comparable statutory measures within the country concerned.

In the British context there is really only one precedent for statutorily required ethical review of research, and once again it may not be sufficiently close for conclusions to be drawn with confidence. The precedent concerns that very particular and special area of research we mentioned in Chapter One, namely research carried out on human embryos. In order to be granted a licence to carry out such research, the relevant institutions must satisfy a statutory authority, the Human Fertilisation and Embryology Authority (HFEA), on its clinical, technical and ethical standards, which include the required establishment and use of institutional RECs[3]. The actual connection between the law and the requirement for REC review is admittedly indirect. The law makes it a criminal offence to conduct research on human embryos without a licence for the specific piece of research in question. The licence can be obtained only from the HFEA, which is legally empowered to set qualifying conditions. These qualifying conditions, set out in its Code of Practice and expressed in the structure of the licence application documents, include the specific requirement that to be licensed, a particular research proposal must have been approved by a properly-constituted ethics committee. In practice, then, to conduct embryo research lawfully you must get a licence from the HFEA, and to get a licence you have to do whatever the HFEA may lawfully require you to do. This currently includes satisfying a process of ethical review. This is, in Britain, as close as one can presently get to an example of statutory ethical review of research. What can we learn from it?

The principal positive effect of this statutory measure is to require that this kind of research be carried out only by practitioners who are competent, properly equipped and responsible, something that would be applauded in the case of clinical research in general. In the context of embryo research it provides substantial reassurance to anyone who thinks that embryo research is a proper thing to do but nevertheless something which must be done within morally important limits and in a responsible and sensitive way. Of course not everyone thinks that human embryo research **is** a proper thing to do if it results – as it frequently does – in denying the embryos in question the possibility of continued life and development. In thinking about what we can learn from the example it is interesting to reflect that one of the elements of disagreement, between those who accept and those who deny that human embryo research is ethically acceptable, concerns our view of what sort of entity the early human embryo actually is. All might agree that it deserves the degree of respect necessary to make sure that embryo research is not conducted in a casual, capricious or self-evidently futile way, nor in a way that would give obvious public offence. But people disagree over whether the embryo deserves to be protected from lethal harm, if the death of the embryo is the price to be paid for clinically valuable knowledge.

As research subjects, then, the official view is that human embryos are not like other human research subjects, something which has important implications for the sorts of protections which we might want to secure through statute. There is no agreement that embryos have the same sorts of interests or deserve the same sort of protections as human subjects in general, and the licensing of embryo research proceeds on the presumption that they do not. Whether or not embryos deserve better, this view is certainly consistent with the position in other relevant matters of the law in England and Wales. Unlike live-born human research subjects, embryos are not protected from battery, from assault, from manslaughter, from murder nor, as embryos, from the results of clinical negligence[4]. But since even the best-regulated research can lawfully undertake actions leading to the destruction of the embryos in question, it could hardly be argued that the statutory regulation of embryo research 'makes up for' deficiencies in other forms of legal protection. What interests then are protected in the regulation of embryo research? At the level of ensuring the competence and expertise of the researchers and facilities, the interests are those of the ultimate beneficiaries of the research, mainly infertile couples. Regulating embryo research makes it more likely that embryology will advance on the basis of reliable data, and less likely that ill-founded and hence hazardous clinical procedures would find their way into wider use. At the level of ethical review, however, the relevant interests are presumably those rather ill-defined interests of public decency. For instance, one of the morally important criteria to be applied in considering proposed embryo research concerns whether it is necessary to carry out the research on live human embryos at all as distinct from some other biological material. If we think this restriction is important, but we also think that when the condition is met then the embryos in question may effectively be put to death in the interests of the knowledge thereby gained, then clearly the interests of the embryos themselves are not thought paramount. Rather, the restriction seems to defend our concern that the embryos be not destroyed needlessly, wantonly or capriciously. It is more plausibly our own consciences than the embryos in question which are protected.

Whilst no-one would deny that these concerns are important also in general clinical research on human subjects, a crucial focus of 'public decency' in this more general context lies in upholding the sort of respect and protection that individual human subjects ought to enjoy. This concern, rather than the clarity of society's conscience, is what drives ethical review. So it seems that both in effect and in underlying intention, the difference between embryo research and general clinical research is profound. As a result, the precedent of the law's involvement in ethical review of embryo research may not offer us much guidance as to the likely effects of putting ethical review of general clinical research on a statutory footing.

It is true, as we noted, that the wider regulation of embryo research tends towards ensuring that it be carried out only by competent and responsible researchers. This would be a good thing in any clinical research context (indeed, in any research context whatever). For embryo research it may be that statutory regulation can achieve more than a merely voluntary system of regulation, such as that which for a while preceded the law establishing the HFEA. Withdrawal of approval from a research project by the body operative at the time, the Voluntary Licensing Authority, made it awkward but not impossible to continue with research that was thought questionable by the Authority. Withdrawal of licence by the HFEA now makes such research impossible within the law. Would the same gain be achieved in wider clinical research? The answer here is probably 'no'. Pharmaceutical research is overwhelmingly supported by the pharmaceutical industry itself, whose veto over industry-funded research is virtually absolute. As regards other kinds of clinical research, in practice the qualifying conditions for obtaining funding, achieving respectable publication, retaining membership of professional bodies and – not least – remaining within the terms of National Health Service employment contracts combine to make ethical approval effectively mandatory. It's therefore not clear what statutory ethical review would add. As we noted at the conclusion of Chapter Ten, the challenge is to make ethical review effective and efficient; the question of whether a statutory basis is really necessary for ethical review is secondary to the question of whether we can make the present system work.

13.2 A wider remit for RECs? The economic implications of innovation

People who like this sort of thing will find this the sort of thing that they like.
(Abraham Lincoln)

Most people accept that there is an inevitable and unbridgeable gap between the demand for health care provision and the availability of the resources needed to service that demand[5]. Since in most industrial countries there has been an historical increase in that proportion of gross national product which is spent on health care[6], then either the absolute level of demand is fairly constant but simply out of reach of any realistic level of resource provision, or health care demand itself grows, continuously staying ahead of growth in resource provision. The second explanation is the accepted one, and part of the continuous growth in health care demand is attributed to the ever-greater expectations people have concerning what medicine can or might be able to do for them[7]. These expectations don't arise in a vacuum; they are largely fuelled by medical technical innovation, whose attendant publicity is part of the staple diet of television news and current affairs. And this gives us a moral problem. For if a shortage in health care resources forces us to make choices between which forms of patient care will receive increased funds and which will not, then we are forced to choose among the competing clinical interests of different individuals. Since this constitutes a morally troubling situation in itself, those pressures that give rise to the situation also require our moral attention.

Specifically, if unfettered medical innovation increases the pressure on health care resources (and we are taking it that it does, through inflating our expectations of what health care could do for us) then even medical innovation which is successful in clinical terms is not the unambiguously good thing that we might otherwise have imagined it to be. This was recognised well before the current spate of National Health Service reforms (which are expressly aimed at keeping health care provision within planned and controlled spending targets). For instance, in what with hindsight was a landmark discussion, Stocking and Morrison identified, and to some extent defended, the possibility that responsible health planning might mean taking steps to avoid the effects of technological advance[8]. Of course if the effects can't easily be detached from the advance in question, then the simplest step is to resist or reject the advance as such, together with any benefits it might have produced. This is an uncomfortable reflection, but one which the economic constraints of modern publicly-funded health care force us to contemplate. In any situation of scarcity, the adoption of one form of provision has 'knock-on' effects on the wider system of provision as a whole, in terms both of initial purchase and continuing staffing, maintenance and replacement costs.

Stocking and Morrison realised that the introduction of new technologies might have to be 'managed' in a way that recognised the possible implications of their future development; in economic terms, the adoption of one technology may mean that another has to be foregone[9].

Since their study of computed tomographic (CT) scanners, more recent clinical innovations have even more graphically illustrated a further way in which technological advance can generate novel demands upon health care resources. The introduction and refinement of *in vitro* fertilisation (IVF) into the previously rather limited range of assisted conception services has not merely responded to a clinical need but has in a very real sense helped to **create** it, by encouraging the conversion of childlessness, a basically social category, into infertility, an essentially medical category that is clinically diagnosable and in many instances 'treatable' (in the limited sense that underlying pathology can be evaded or cheated, although not cured). The essential point is the same, however, in the case of both CT scanners and IVF; the more that technology enables us to do, the more demand is created. Stocking and Morrison noticed that this is true amongst both patients and their doctors who, in particular, may be tempted to believe that greater precision in diagnosis is always necessary and beneficial, and that a readily available CT scanner should become 'one more test .... which the patient must have'[10] (incidentally further adding to the technological emphasis of modern health care, within which subsequent technical innovations will be expected). These specific demands are superimposed upon the existing pattern of health care demand, in the process changing its centre of gravity. Nowhere is this more true than in the case of diagnostic technology like the CT scanner, whose introduction improved the detection of progressive diseases ever before it could stimulate improved therapy. Inevitably it drove further demands on the part of clinical practitioners for screening programmes and on the part of patients for more research into better therapeutic measures against the diseases being detected. Of course, early detection could lead to improvements in treatment outcomes and hence, in principle, to the freeing of resources previously tied up in extensive surgery and the eventual management of the end-stages of terminal disease: but this cannot be assumed. Indeed, part of the problem of knowing how to respond to the additional demands generated by technological innovation is the fact that, without good data on the effects which the new technologies actually have on treatment outcomes, the technologies cannot themselves be properly evaluated either clinically or economically. As Stocking and Morrison complained, the outcome assessment which is taken for granted in pharmaceutical development was largely missing from other areas of medical innovation at the time of their study (1978)[11]; the situation has not essentially changed since then.

However, suppose that usable clinical data **were** available from preliminary studies on specific diagnostic and other technical innovations, much in the same way as Phase III pharmaceutical studies proceed on the basis of data from preliminary studies. Suppose that for a given innovation – say a particular diagnostic use of a CT scanner – there were good data to show that the equipment could demonstrate a certain disease condition with equal success and with far less risk or discomfort than the current standard method (perhaps surgical biopsy). Suppose finally that it is proposed to undertake a large study of whether equally good results can be obtained over a wide range of patients, with a larger number of clinical operators, and perhaps in connection with other disease conditions at a comparably early stage of pathological development; such a study would naturally come to an REC for ethical review. On the account put forward by Stocking and Morrison, an assessment of the technology's clinical success is only part of the picture. As they put it:

> …when a technology is evaluated it is not enough to compare its usefulness with that of another technology or another form of health care now. Explicit recognition must be given to the effects of future developments and arrangements for continuing evaluation and assessment of the technology must be made as these developments take place.[12]

or, more succinctly, '…technology must be assessed not only for its clinical efficacy but also for its effects on the system in which it operates'[13]. The costs of the introduction of a new technology will be paid in terms of those effects, including having to give up the alternative uses to which those resources committed to the new technology would otherwise have been put. The economic implications of innovation are real, and must be faced.

Before considering how this might be done, and who ought to do it, we should recognise just how uncomfortable such considerations are, morally speaking. If the innovation has any clinical value then, whether the innovation be adopted or rejected, someone or other will be denied the clinical benefit that they would otherwise have obtained. As we saw when we considered the conflicting interests at stake in clinical research (see section 2.1) we have to counterbalance the interests of those who are sick now against the interests of those who might become sick in the future. It is tempting to think that our existing obligations to the presently ill must be stronger than our conjectured or hypothetical future obligations concerning what we might one day be able to do for other, as yet unknown, people who might one day be ill. We might well want to give 'moral primacy' to the patients who are in front of us now and for whose benefit we can commit known quantities of present resources[14]. The trouble with this supposition is that it is usually unrealistic to separate present and future patients in this way, particularly when the innovation in question concerns developments or refinements to the investigation and management of conditions to which resources are already being committed. Innovations which 'create' new classes of patients (an example might be the micro-manipulation of immotile sperm, making possible the 'treatment' of male factor infertility) are comparatively very rare. This of course does not really answer the point about the primacy of present moral obligations; rather it avoids it, though perhaps fairly. Another way of avoiding the point is to recall that technical innovation might in fact lead to savings in health care resources, thus increasing the pool available for future expenditure and thereby serving the interests of both present and future patients across different disease categories. Again this is a fair response but of course it is one which relies on an explicit appeal to the resource impact of the innovation, and which thereby confirms that the impact of innovations must be studied in economic as well as clinical terms.

If there is a good case for thinking that these impacts should be studied, who should study them? In discussing the wider impact of the CT scanner, Stocking and Morrison identified a wide range of relevant groups and effects, and defended them all as being relevant to the assessment of the introduction and use of the new technology. Beginning with the impacts that were then current, that is to say already visible, they noted benefits in terms of the diagnosis and management of patients, but suspected a relatively limited impact on patient outcomes; they distinguished a reinforcement of the emphasis on high technology in the shaping of NHS care; they identified the possible emergence of sub-specialisms within the professional staff associated with using the equipment; they noted pressure on the resource planners within the health service; and they confirmed the reinforcement of current trends in research and development within the British medical/technical industry[15]. More provocatively, they considered the likely changes in all these effects in the event of various possible future scenarios, such as a significant fall in the unit price of scanners; developments in the diagnostic capabilities of the equipment; the development of effective therapies for the cancers being diagnosed; and general improvements in other forms of medical imaging technologies[16]. In each case the then-current impacts had to be reassessed, and whilst in some instances they were confirmed or reinforced, in other cases the impacts were reversed. Interestingly, the impact on patient outcomes – already regarded as relatively limited in the (then) short term – was also the least affected by the different eventualities they considered. Far greater variations (including adverse effects) were to be found in the impacts upon NHS planners, upon the shape of the NHS and the pattern of demand for care, and upon the relevant sector of British industry[17]! Perhaps a technology which is predicted to have more impact in these areas than on patients' disease outcomes is a particularly good candidate for economic as well as clinical evaluation. And perhaps such a technology is the exception rather than the rule in medical innovation. But even to find out whether it is exceptional, we need the sort of combined clinical and socio-economic data on which the assessments conducted, defended and commended by Stocking and Morrison are based.

For our present purposes it is probably simplest to concede the importance of this kind of impact-assessment of new technology, but to acknowledge at the same time that it must rely on socio-economic competencies that lie well outside those normally to be expected within the structures of clinical ethical review. This is inevitable – but it is frustrating and unsatisfactory as well, because the economic implications of specific innovations are certainly relevant to the ethical review of their development. As we noted when we considered the problem of multiple research objectives (in section 3.4) and the recruitment of volunteers to Phase I pharmaceutical research (in section 6.4) the future prospects of a new product or device hold the key to whether or not there is any point to current testing. If it could reliably be foreseen that the economic cost of an innovation would prevent its further development then we would know that current stages of research were futile: and we have agreed that it is unethical to expose research subjects to pointless risk. In other words, if an REC had a crystal ball then they would plainly be obliged to inspect it when reviewing current research protocols. Since crystal balls are notoriously unavailable even in the private sector, then ethical review of research would have much to gain from more formalised assessment of the impact of new technologies and products.

13.3   From research to practice: the hospital ethics committee?

I can't stand whispering. Every time a doctor whispers
in the hospital, next day there's a funeral.
(Neil Simon)

Unlike a number of other countries, notably the United States[18], Britain has no accepted tradition of ethical review of clinical practice, although there are individual hospital ethics committees that do consider issues arising from practice rather than research[19] and the idea is gaining a certain amount of currency. The ethical review of clinical practice differs from that of clinical research in several important respects, basically mirroring key differences between practice and research themselves. It is worth our while considering these differences.

First, there is the difference that has occupied us throughout this book: that research, unlike practice, is primarily concerned with promoting interests other than those of the patient presently before us. Connectedly, there has to be a more systematic character to research than the 'trial and error' empiricism appropriate to practice. Protocols are designed to exclude unwanted variables, and typically they require a cohort of human subjects who are as alike as possible in terms of the key variables; for this purpose exclusion criteria will screen out people who don't fit. Practice, on the other hand, is essentially about understanding and responding to those differences among individuals that underlie and transform their particular experiences of ill-health. In these respects, the more detached, impersonal character of research distances the researcher from the welfare of the research subject in a way that demands compensating protections of the kind intended by ethical review. By contrast, clinical practice flourishes best in a mutual understanding and involvement between clinician and patient. If it is natural to see the need for ethical review of impersonal clinical arrangements, it seems correspondingly natural also to stand aside from the intimacy of the clinical practice encounter.

Another way of looking at this is to recognise that clinical research is a special sort of departure from clinical practice. The centre of gravity of clinical medicine lies in the personal clinical encounters between doctor and patient. (As we have noted already, if this is a romantic view of clinical medicine it is also a widespread and durable one, and it enables us to explore the contrast between research and practice.) Clinical research deliberately abstracts from these encounters everything that makes them into individual relationships. Whilst there is something in the argument that the standards of consent required in clinical practice should be 'levelled up' to match those of clinical research, if there is to be a difference between those standards then it certainly ought to favour the research context, where the patient we might say journeys alone rather than in the company of his physician. It follows from all of this that what is clearly a protection in the case of research can too easily appear to be an intrusion in the case of practice: if it is appropriate to oversee the way the research subject is identified, enrolled and conducted through a series of events not designed for his express benefit, it can seem inappropriate to apply the same scrutiny to the way that an ordinary patient is individually accompanied through a series of events cast so far as is possible in his individual interests.

These observations should make us cautious about the case for ethical review of practice; they should not, however, incline us to reject it out of hand. Here are some arguments in favour of the idea of hospital ethics committees looking at issues arising from clinical practice. First, in connection with individual clinical relationships, we should recognise that the moral dimensions of clinical responsibility are not unique, mysterious or private. Patients need reassurance and perhaps redress if things go wrong, and there is a transparent public interest in mechanisms to provide them. Patients are vulnerable; they can make mistakes and they can be overwhelmed by their circumstances. Clinicians too can make mistakes; and they are not saints and they should not be expected to have infinite insight or tolerance. Moreover, clinicians themselves might want to be protected from some of the burdens of too-extensive moral responsibility: a 'neutral' source of support and counsel would help them whilst offering indirect benefits to their patients. The increasing use of team-based care and of high-tech machinery for diagnosis are in any case diluting the one-to-one clinical relationship of old, certainly restricting and perhaps even defeating it in extreme cases such as that of the Intensive Therapy Unit. And innovations in clinical practice produce novel moral situations or obligations, for instance as in the case of pleas to withdraw hydration and nutrition from those who nowadays survive catastrophic brain damage[20].

Second, and arising from these last considerations, concerns arising in individual clinical situations often generate questions of wider policy: clinical ethics, like scientific medicine, proceeds by generalising individual experiences as well as by bringing prior (and wider) understanding to the present problem. The emergent need for protocols to define the management of patients in clinical problem areas[21] echoes a need for something else as well, more personal and less remote than a printed document: a neutral court of counsel where those carrying clinical responsibility can formally share it and reflect on it. At the very least, on this view, a body such as a hospital ethics committee offers a middle road between individualist clinical autonomy and slavish adherence to external mechanisms such as protocols.

Arguments against the establishment of hospital ethics committees are primarily aimed at the version which has such committees pronouncing judgement on individual clinical cases rather than providing a forum for general evolution of difficult areas of practice. The most prominent of these arguments is simply that the sanctity of the clinical relationship should not be intruded upon; in plausible support, it objects that even a committee composed exclusively of relevant professionals, all of whom were well accustomed to carrying precisely the kind of clinical responsibility in question, could not know the patient as he is known by his personal doctor. (Heaven forfend, therefore, that we should take our problems to a wider body of whom some were laymen in medical terms...) This is of course an appeal to the clinical prerogative – which is usually cited in terms of the paternalist's withholding of information when judged in the patient's interest, but is here generalised in such a manner as to resist ethical review even by the professional peer group. The appeal can be rebutted, of course, because the very assumption that the clinician should be the final judge of the patient's interests is in itself a potent issue for ethical review in the research context. In attempting to subdue wider ethical concern, the appeal to the clinical prerogative serves only to stimulate it. However, stripped of the appeal, there is still clearly a charge to be answered in the matter of intrusion into a relationship for which someone else carries responsibility. A concomitant danger, if that intrusion became routine, is that clinicians would begin by resenting it and end by relying on it. Some years ago the authors learned – at first hand from one of the professionals involved – of how far this intrusion can damage the traditional clinical relationship: a severely mentally-handicapped girl sustained additional (and in the end lethal) brain damage in a fall. Apparently fearing the consequences of taking clinical responsibility more than those of relinquishing it, the attending physician arranged to have the girl put on a ventilator **in order to** enable the convening of a meeting of the ethics committee[22].

Against the more modest conception, of a hospital ethics committee which reviews only general issues arising out of clinical practice, there are more modest objections. Principally, would such committees encourage too-early resort to things like protocols, thereby contributing to the gradual de-personalisation of clinical care? It seems hardly less speculative to deny this than it is to allege it: it would at any rate be the responsibility of such review bodies to keep their reflections as close as possible to the individuality of clinical work without intruding on its intimacy, and that might be no easy matter. The complementary guise of this objection is to point to the opposite danger: that, once established, hospital ethics committees would find it increasingly difficult to remain detached from individual clinical cases, and to resist the temptation to become involved in specific individual clinical judgements (at which point the balance of the lay and professional membership becomes more delicate than ever). Whatever the intentions, so this objection goes, intrusion into the clinical relationship is inevitable. All one can say is, again, that the danger is a real one and can be avoided only by the responsible self-restraint of the ethics committee. Confining individual cases to use as illustrations of general issues rather than as occasions for specific peer intervention can preserve the privacy and sanctity of the individual clinical relationship – but it would be a stiff challenge to the prudence and humility of those involved in the review process, and perhaps no less stiff for the lay members than for the clinical professionals.

13.4   Ethical review of health policy? A case example

> *The longer I practise medicine the more convinced I am that there are only two types of cases: those that involve taking the trousers off and those that don't.*
> (Alan Bennett)

Since in this chapter we are engaged in a little crystal-ball-gazing ourselves, let us return for a moment to the crystal ball we referred to previously, unfortunately not available to RECs, concerning the socio-economic impact of new therapies. We have agreed that RECs generally lack the competencies need to carry out a proper assessment of that impact, but we also recognised that if the exercise were carried out by a competent authority elsewhere then an REC would be obliged to consider the assessment as relevant. A parallel consideration is that it is not merely the outcomes but also the processes of clinical research which have social and economic impact.

Clinical research is a large industry; taking part in it earns professional and academic prestige amongst clinicians; its objects and methods help to drive health care demand and hence, if only by default, health policy; and time spent by clinical carers in research activity is only (and at best) coincidentally time spent in clinical care itself; even the best-designed protocols confer upon the subjects of research an artificial uniformity which does not really belong in individual clinical care. Indeed, the distribution of clinical time between practice and research is in Britain an emergent issue for management, particularly in the case of the newly-independent health care management trusts; the REC's position as advisory committees to management accordingly becomes somewhat delicate[23]. Research is of course only one factor in planning health policy, but it is a significant and visible one; and when research is made subject to health policy then ethical review itself becomes, for management, merely part of a wider assessment.

But of course this should serve simply to remind us that health policy itself has enormous ethical implications: why should not these in their turn also be reviewed formally? If the case is made for ethical review of the economic implications of particular items of research (and of the practices to which they are likely to give rise), then should we not generalise the case: should we not undertake ethical review of the socio-economic implications of entire health policies – of present patterns of provision as well as of those conjectured patterns which could arise from adopting novel methods/procedures piecemeal? Clearly if the more limited case is beyond the competence of the standard REC then this more ambitious programme is doubly so. But if we accept the aim, then must accept the case for finding the means.

Arguments could be mounted against the aim. Recall our attempt to counterpose our obligations to the currently ill and our obligations to the future beneficiaries of research. No-one is compelled to accept that making health policies and their socio-economic implications visible, non-arbitrary, rational and pro-active is better than retaining an *ad hoc*, reactive approach to health policy, allowing its implications to remain unexplored for fear of taking long-range decisions which visibly, cold-bloodedly and systematically discriminate against those groups from whom future marginal resources will knowingly be withdrawn (or, more soothingly, 'disinvested'). And whilst most of us might be tempted to think that rationality is finally better than '*ad hock*ery' it's salutary to remember that, if we were really concerned only with producing most health care per pound spent, then we would put all our resources into an extended form of accident and emergency care geared to getting the reversibly sick back to their places of work. In a sense, only moral reasons underlie our conviction that health care is more than this.

Ironically, this last observation began as an argument against the aim of a systematic review of health policy. As such it's a spectacular failure, because it effectively demonstrates the need for assessing health policy in the light of ethical concerns, of which the extension of health care to the non-productive sectors of the population is clearly one. Let us then accept the case for ethical review of health policy, and conclude by noting an example of an ethical review committee established to do just that. One of the Welsh District Health Authorities, namely that in West Glamorgan, in 1993 established a 'Local Ethics Committee (Purchaser Advice)' to provide explicitly ethical review of resource planning and health policy[24]. The Committee is an advisory body only and its refusal to endorse a planning or policy proposal does not obstruct the Health Authority's going ahead – in this sense it is less powerful than the corresponding REC, since the Department of Health's *Guidelines* expressly instruct Health Authorities not to permit research which does not enjoy ethical approval. There is no such provision regarding the advice of the 'Purchaser Advice' committee, which is of course a novel phenomenon. However the Health Authority has decided to submit all its spending plans to the Purchaser Advice Committee for ethical review. The most significant aspect of this seems to be the recognition on the part of a Health Authority that all of its planning decisions have 'inescapably moral elements'[25]. (It is too early to know whether the Committee's advice will make a difference to the Authority's decisions, or if so what kind of effect this will be[26].) The membership of the Committee appears somewhat to resemble that of any local REC[27]. This suggests that the Committee's brief does not extend into the kind of formal socio-economic impact assessment we considered above; such assessments would form a natural part of the evidence which the Committee could consider, though its competencies as presently conducted seem to be continuous with those deployed in the ethical review of research.

This is not yet an expansion of the rôle of the REC; it is however an expansion of the **idea** of ethical review. In this book we have been concerned to explore that idea, its requirements and its implications. The West Glamorgan initiative reminds us that the implications of ethical review extend beyond clinical research itself, but it is in the field of clinical research that ethical review has come of age. Ethical review is now accepted and respected as an integral part of pursuing effective and responsible research. Perhaps in the future it will similarly be seen as integral to the responsible provision of health care as well, at the level both of recurrent clinical practice and of health policy.

Notes

1   The most important to date is European Commission Directive No. 91/507/EEC, dated 19th July 1991.

2   Personal communication from Dr Søren Holm, University of Cophenhagen.

3   Human Fertilisation and Embryology Authority: *Code of Practice*, London: HFEA (1993, revised), para. 9.6.

4   The law of negligence provides for individuals to sue in respect of negligent harms they suffered *in utero*; but in order to do so they must have been born alive and hence this redress is not available to embryos destined for research rather than for implantation and gestation. Presumably there could be **other** plaintiffs in a case of negligence arising from the treatment or use of so-called 'research embryos', for instance whoever at the time holds the legal title to 'disposal' of the embryos. We are grateful to Richard Townshend-Smith for this information.

5   For instance, see Drummond, M.F., *Principles of Economic Appraisal in Health Care*, Oxford University Press (1980) p. 2.

6   For instance in the United Kingdom the proportion of Gross National Product (GNP) spent on health care was 4.1% in 1950, 5.5% in 1976 and 6.1% in 1983, falling to 5.8% in 1991. Appleby, J., *Financing health care in the 1990s*, Buckingham: Open University Press (1992).

7   For a discussion of this problem and its implications see Evans, M., 'The "management" of demand for Health Care', *International Journal of Health Care Quality Assurance*, 3:2 (1990), pp. 5-10.

8   Stocking, B. and Morrison, S.L., *The Image and the Reality: a Case Study of the Impacts of Medical Technology*, London/Oxford: Nuffield Provincial Hospitals Trust/Oxford University Press, (1978). On page 50 they say: '...in looking at potential impacts it may be that responsible bodies may wish to take steps to make sure the impacts suggested do **not** come about.' [original emphasis].

9   Stocking and Morrison, *op.cit.*, p. 2.

10 Stocking & Morrison, *op. cit.*, p. 56.

11 *op. cit.*, p. 62.

12 *ibid.*, p. 4.

13 *ibid.*, pp. 64/5.

14 This point is explored rather further in Evans, M., *op. cit.*, pp. 5-10.

15 Current and future hypothetical impacts are succinctly tabulated in Stocking and Morrison, *op. cit.*, pp. 48/9.

16 *ibid.*

17 *ibid.*

18 In the U.S.A., the term 'ethics committee' standardly denotes a body reviewing practice, as distinct from research where the relevant committees are known instead as Institutional Review Boards (IRBs).

19 For instance, the John Radcliffe Hospital in Cambridge has such a committee.

20 The much-discussed case of Anthony Bland, the young man five years in the persistent vegetative state, raised general issues of policy as well as of practice. See Andrews, K., 'Patients in the persistent vegetative state: problems in their long-term management', *British Medical Journal* 306

214 · · · The future of ethical review

(1993), pp. 1600-1602; and, *contra*, Gillon, R., 'Patients in the persistent vegetative state: a response to Dr. Andrews', *loc. cit.*, pp. 1602-1603.

21 Consider, for instance, the problems of knowing in advance when not to treat premature and very low birth weight babies, or of deciding whether it is appropriate to move a dying patient from a general medical ward to an ITU in order to enable them to serve as an organ donor.

22 We are grateful to Professor Larry Heintz of the University of Hawaii for this example.

23 An REC known to the authors has been forced to evolve a policy on responding to management requests for information about those applications received by the REC from clinicians employed by the relevant authorities. The overlap between information for planning resource policy and information on employees' working practices is uncomfortably broad.

24 Jarvis, R., 'Health care planning: an ethical dimension?', *Bulletin of Medical Ethics*, 95 (1994): pp. 17-18.

25 Jarvis, *op. cit.*, p.18.

26 Jarvis is to pursue these very questions in his work as Research Scholar, a post funded by the Authority in part to service the Purchaser Advice Committee; *ibid.*

27 *ibid.*, p. 17.

Index

Index compiled by INDEXING SPECIALISTS.

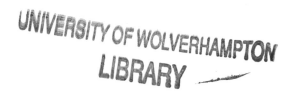

Wiley Titles of Related Interest...

RESEARCH IN HEALTH CARE
Design, Conduct and Interpretation of Health Services Research
I. CROMBIE with H.T.O. DAVIES

An accessible and jargon-free guide which meets the urgent need for practical advice on the design, conduct, analysis and interpretation of research. Providing a basis for health care policy and planning, it addresses a medical area which is experiencing rapid expansion

0471 96259 7   312pp   1996   Paperback

PRIORITY SETTING: THE HEALTH CARE DEBATE
Edited by J. COAST, J. DONOVAN and S. FRANKEL

Critically analyses the issues raised by health care rationing and details the policy options available. A comprehensive guide to policy, offering practical tips and information, it pointedly examines the issues of health economics, epidemiology and medical ethics.
0471 96102 7   296pp   1996

PRINCIPLES OF HEALTH CARE ETHICS
Edited by R. GILLON and A. LLOYD

Over 100 authors, representing a wide range of disciplines, nationalities and cultures, discuss the many complex ethical dilemmas posed by modern medicine and health care in this richly diverse and thought-provoking collection.

"...an invaluable and lasting contribution to the ever-changing and controversial topic of health care ethics."

Journal of the Royal College of Physicians

0471 93033 4   1152pp   1993

Journals from Wiley...

HEALTH CARE ANALYSIS
Journal of Health Philosophy and Policy
Editor: D. SEEDHOUSE

Carries analysis of fundamental issues in health care and policy and provides clarification of current theories, investigating their effects on policy and practice.
ISSN: 1065-3058   Quarterly